Social Work in the Hospital Organization

Love can not fill the thickened lung with breath,
Nor clean the blood, nor set the fractured bone;
Yet many a man is making friends with death
Even as I speak, for lack of love alone.

Edna St.Vincent Millay,
Sonnet xxx, in *Fatal Interview*
Collected Sonnets of
Edna St.Vincent Millay (Harper & Row).

Social Work
in the
Hospital
Organization

MARGARET GAUGHAN BROCK

University of Toronto Press

© University of Toronto Press 1969
Reprinted 1971
ISBN 0-8020-1594-8
LC 71-382829
Printed in Canada

The lines facing the title-page are from Sonnet
XXX of *Fatal Interview; Collected Poems*, Harper & Row, Copyright 1931, 1958, by Edna St.
Vincent Millay and Norma Millay Ellis. By
permission of Norma Millay Ellis.

CONTENTS

ACKNOWLEDGMENTS

Many people helped me to write this book, people I have known and worked with through long years: patients and co-workers of every profession and staff members from every department in the hospital. I thank them all. With the exception of several worthwhile years in a family agency, all my professional experience has been in a medical setting where I have worked on all services and with doctors who included chiefs, attending staff, residents and interns, as well as nurses in all categories from director to beginning students. I have worked in Montreal, Quebec, Hagerstown, Maryland and Toronto, Ontario, and although each community was unique, each was also the same because of the great and wonderful communality of mankind.

A few people I want to thank particularly. Many, by both precept and example, taught me what dynamic administration could be and the late Dr. Perry Prather, former Director of Health, Maryland State Department of Health, showed me that policies and regulations are guide lines only, which, if they interfere with obtaining help for a patient, should be considered flexible. Mrs. Josephine Chaisson, with whom I have shared so much that has made both life and social work exciting, encouraged and advised in the presentation of the material. Others encouraged too: Miss Jeri Cohn and Miss Lily Duchess, both members of my staff, cheered all the way. Miss Francess Halpenny of the Press, who read the manuscript, earned my gratitude for her understanding and patience. There would have been no manuscript without my secretary, Mrs. Christina Chobrzynski, who struggled with my illegible writing and typed and re-typed, always with interest and enthusiasm. All my students in social work, hospital administration and nursing made me realize, gratefully, that a teacher is also taught. Much of my experience coalesced and was tested while I was Director of Social Work, New Mount Sinai Hospital, Toronto, but this would not have been possible without the support of the Board under the chairmanship of Mr. Ben Sadowski, Mr. Gurston S. Allen, first chairman of the Social Service Committee, and the understanding and support of the Administrator (now Executive Director), Mr. Sidney Liswood.

Social Work in the Hospital Organization

CHAPTER I

INTRODUCTION

This book was written for those interested in having
a basic text about medical social work. The material
has specific reference to social work in the hospital
organization, but much of it is applicable to social
work within the broader context of health care. It
is a crystallization of my experience of twenty-five
years as a medical social worker, not only in practice but also as a supervisor and teacher; it undoubtedly also reflects many concepts that I have
over the years encountered in the work of others and
no longer recognize as being the result of reading
an uncountable number of books and articles on the
subject. All such debts, conscious and unconscious,
are acknowledged with gratitude.

Any printed material now available on establishing and administering social work in the hospital
organization is largely incidental reference in a
multitude of books and articles; it may often appear
without adequate context so that it serves to confuse
rather than to enlighten. The unfortunate consequence
is that students in hospital administration, social
work, nursing, and in some universities, medicine,
may have inadequate knowledge of the subject, and
will find an assignment on the topic of social work
in the health field a frustrating experience. This
book has their needs in mind also. Perhaps, too, it
will be of help to members of hospital boards and
hospital administrators who wish to establish a
social service department or evaluate one already in
operation. Indeed, most of the material to be presented has already been tested by a number of individuals working in the areas just mentioned.

Certainly, this book does not try to exhaust
the subject. Moreover, some administrators, doctors,
and social workers will undoubtedly find that it
contains points on which they will be pleased to dis-
agree. That is good. Their experience may well be
different from mine. Discussion is healthy and should
be helpful to all, especially to me.

Social work is a professional discipline that is included in those hospital organizations where the hospital authority recognizes that social problems may well be an aspect of illness itself. The primary responsibility of social work is to provide treatment within the area of competence and professional responsibility of the social worker for those patients and their families who require such treatment to help them resolve or effect an adjustment in a social dysfunction that is caused or made more disabling because of illness or hospitalization or both. In some communities social work has been incorporated into the hospital therapeutic program since 1905, but there are still some among whom may be board members, administrators, doctors, and some social workers who question its right to be there. "Patient" may normally be thought of as a label for people who are sick physically, but illness may well have social implications. A hospital authority which wishes to discharge a responsibility to the patient and the community to give total care will therefore require someone in the hospital organization to treat the social pathology; that someone is the social worker. Personnel of all the other professional disciplines have as their first concern their own professional focus, and the social worker in turn takes as her primary concern the intimate and individual social need of the patient. The absence of social service can very well mean a lowering of the quality of patient care.

Social work in the hospital cannot be comprehended without some understanding of social work itself. Chapters on social work are included here but they do not pretend to be definitive; the purpose of this book is not, of course, to teach or discuss the how of doing social work. Its purpose is limited to a discussion of the role and function of social work as it is carried on in a hospital.

The policies and procedures of a social service department postulated in this book are offered as a standard of measurement and not as an absolute. How many of them can or should be put into operation will depend on many variables including the size of the hospital, its geographic location, and its wider community. The decisions are not necessarily dependent on money. However, where professional criteria are involved, the minimum of professional performance cannot and need not be compromised.

This is a mundane book, a record of fact that is offered as an invitation for reflection to those establishing a social service department in a hospital organization. C.A. Mace in <u>The Psychology of Study</u> (Pelican, p. 17) has a description which fits the purpose I have had in mind: "Even an inspired book requires a source of inspiration. Mundane books are either records of fact or of reflection upon fact. The former draw our attention to the facts, the latter invite us to reflect upon the facts for themselves."

CHAPTER II

PROLOGUES HAVE BEEN WRITTEN

"In the continual remembrance of a glorious
past, individuals and nations find their
noblest inspiration, and if to-day this
inspiration so valuable for its own sake,
so important in its associations, is weak-
ened, is it not because in the strong domi-
nance of the individual, so characteristic
of a democracy, we have lost the sense of
continuity?" [1]

From the beginning of recorded time, we are aware
that human beings have cared for other human beings
in some fashion, recognizing the need for help of
those in physical or social distress. Historically,
the motives for giving care and the kind and quality
of care have ranged over a wide spectrum. Assistance
may have been inspired even by the desire for self-
preservation; at the other end of the scale it might
be given because of a love of human beings motivated
by a love of God. Often fear has been the influence
that forced men to make provision for others; often
too it has had a kindlier source. If motives have
varied, so too have the factors that determined both
the quality and the quantity of care throughout history. For example, the economics of the times and
the characteristics of a culture have been significant always in influencing developments. An agrarian
society is less able to provide help in the form of
funds than a technological one. Understanding of
illness or poverty has varied greatly depending on
whether or not mysticism and/or superstition were
characteristics of cultures. The amount of actual
knowledge, not only known but available for knowing,
was obviously a determinant. The amount and kinds
of care given people in any culture, undoubtedly,

---

1. Sir William Osler, *Aequanimitas* (3rd ed.,
Philadelphia, 1945), p. 75.

is likely to be affected also by the degree to which
that culture accepts democracy and respects the dignity and inherent rights of the individual. (The abun-
dance of services which the Soviet Republics provide
for their people reflects perhaps more their value to
the program of the state than a concern for the individual.) Even to-day, it has been known that a city
welfare department denied help because the city fathers believed that the sick and the poor were worth-
less charges and not because of insufficient funds.[2]
This attitude may be contrasted with, for example, the
announcement by the Government of Ontario on March 21,
1967, that as of April 1, 1967, new and flexible regulations for individuals and families receiving assistance would become effective. This legislation, the
Family Benefits Act, operates in conjunction with the
federal government's Canada Assistance Plan and
amounts of financial aid will be determined by actual
financial need.

But though, for many centuries, the care of the
sick and the poor has had some kind of recognition in
one or other of many forms, the structure and methods
of this care have not been well documented. Broad
trends and attitudes and some of the sociological de-
terminants may be visible, but the many streams
through the centuries and the multitude of cultures
that have combined to produce hospitals and social
welfare as they exist to-day have not been adequately
traced. Librarians and authorities in hospital and
social work fields are thus unable to recommend a definitive history of either. Much has been written
about specific periods or particular hospitals or individual methods or areas of social work, but any
attempt to obtain a broad and continuous history of
either hospital or social work finds itself among
fragments. The following sketchy histories have had

2. In 1961, the City Fathers of Newburgh, N.Y., adopt-
ed measures against those in need so punitive that
the New York State Board of Social Welfare intervened.
Various newspapers across the country picked up the
story as lead news. For a social work discussion of
the situation see Samuel Mencher, "Newburgh: The Recurrent Crisis of Public Assistance," in the Journal
of Social Work, published by the National Association
of Social Workers (95 Madison Ave., New York 16),
Vol.7, No.1 (Jan. 1962), p.3.

to be garnered from many sources; they are meant only as a background. [3]

HOSPITALS
     The treatment of disease and the practice of medicine existed long before hospitals. Frequent references are made to methods of caring for the sick and to the maintenance of health in the Old Testament, and references are also found on Egyptian papyri and in early Indian and Greek writings. The first established date of a hospital, according to the sacred books of Thoth, is in Egypt in 4100 B.C. It is believed that during and immediately following this period, hospitals existed in India and Babylon. Apparently they were established in Ceylon by 437 B.C., and in India by 226 B.C., and some understanding of the need to give the sick "tender loving care" was recognized in their policies along with the attention paid to mysticism and superstition. Positive documentation about the period before 500 B.C. is scanty, but during the Golden Age of Greece there is a record of hospitals where not only care of the sick was provided, but refuge was given to the troubled. In the temple of Aesculapius the "sick were ministered to in soul and body." [4] These aesculapia or hospitals were much in the nature of the modern spas, although in many of them treatment and care were given only under the orders and the supervision of a physician. Some had a service comparable to the later day outpatient departments. Teaching was also a common function, influenced by the doctrine of Hippocrates (450-345 B.C.) who taught that disease was a reaction of the body to stress and that treatment was two-fold, physical and social. During the triumphal days of

---

3. Librarians who were consulted could not suggest any particular volume on the history of the hospital development. From Charity to Social Work by Kathleen Woodroofe, published by Routledge and Kegan Paul, London, and University of Toronto Press in North America is most informative on the history of social work. Attention must be drawn to the fact that this book relates only to England and the United States.

4. Malcolm T. MacEachern, Hospital Organization and Management (2nd ed., Chicago, 1947), p. 3.

the Roman Empire, physical fitness was a supreme
asset; the fighting man especially was important and
resources were provided to restore him to the fray.
The word nosocomia was used to denote these institutions.

With the spread of the Gospel of Christ and the
preachings of St. Paul, the concept of charity (meaning love) was born. With this base, the care of the
sick, the poor, and the needy took on a fresh meaning, and hospitals were founded as an act of piety
and as a charitable endeavour. For centuries, these
motives continued to be the stimuli for the construc-
tion of hospitals, institutions that were to become
the modern hospitals as we know them. Perhaps the
first of these was built in Caesarea, in Cappodocia,
in 369 A.D., when St. Basil was bishop. The first
hospital in Europe was in Rome, a monument to the
charity and piety of the holy woman Fabiola; she was
one of a group of high-born Roman ladies who dedicated
their lives to caring for the sick and the unfortunate. Both St. Basil and Fabiola were clear in stating
the aims of their institutions: to give care to the
sick, the aged and the orphans. As the years passed
and other men and women founded monasteries and con-
gregations, more facilities for the care of the people
in physical and social difficulties became available.
Indeed, in their Rule, most religious orders included
an obligation to provide a room not only for their
own sick members but for the troubled transient, the
sick and the weary. However, during the early part of
the Middle Ages the standards of human beings, then
as now, were open to change, and history records not
only a levelling off but a deterioration in standards
of care. The Crusaders who from 1066 to 1270 fought
the Holy Wars far from home needed attention for their
wounds, and perhaps for homesickness; they established
infirmaries along their routes of travel. The Hôtel
Dieu was established in Paris in 660 A.D.; St. John's
at York was built in 1084. Thus there are records of
isolated attempts to provide adequate attention for
the poor and the ill, but there was no real and last-
ing development.

With the first awakenings of the Renaissance,
St. Bartholomew's was founded in London in 1177, and
it has remained a most notable hospital. By the beginning of the late 1500's, there is evidence that care

improved, knowledge increased and was formally taught.
The population as a whole began to take some responsibility for the care of the sick and the poor, and
although in many countries the religious orders continued to give leadership it was no longer solely in
the hands of the monks and the clerics. In 1633, the
Order of the Daughters of Charity of St. Vincent de
Paul was established in France, a prototype of a nursing service.

Until the end of the eighteenth century, records
of conditions in hospitals, judged by our standards
were frightful. Several patients occupied one bed, [5]
often a pallet on the floor; cleanliness, which had
been important in ancient times, was forgotten and
suppuration was believed to be the body trying to
heal itself. It usually did by death, but not before
infection and disease had spread. When the explorers
and immigrants came to the brave New World of North
America, they brought their culture with them. Therefore it is not surprising to learn that Cortez founded a hospital in Mexico City in 1520, just twenty-
eight years after the voyage of Columbus. Quebec in
1639 and Montreal in 1644 had institutions for the
care and protection of their sick, and in British
North America, New York in 1736 and Philadelphia in
1751 established well-known hospitals that today are
still giving care with standards among the highest
in the world.

Beginning in the nineteeth century, the development and growth of hospitals and, indeed, of all methods of giving service to people are better documented.
Knowledge, experience and opportunity, developing
rapidly, were given new momentum by technology, and
technology and scientific advancement are ever increasing forces today. Many men and women made this
possible by their scientific discoveries, by the development of skills and techniques, by the growth of the
nursing profession, above all by the more general dis-
semination of knowledge. Even so, in the early part
of the twentieth century "poor houses" were still
used as a refuge for the aged, the poor and often the
sick, and the tales told of the abuse of the inmates

----

5. In 1964, in Hong Kong hospital wards, two patients
often occupied one bed with two more in cots under
the bed. (Eye witness account by Josephine Chaisson,
personal communication).

by the overseers are at times frightening and at
others pathetic. The poem, later set to music, which
was popular in the early 1900's, "Over the Hill to
the Poor House," [6] may seem pathetic today but perhaps reflects a genuine dread.

In this last half of the twentieth century, hospitals are everywhere and are considered the fifth
largest business on the North America continent. [7]
Of all kinds and all sizes, they contain a proliferation of services and equipment that would startle anyone from the nineteenth century who might visit them.
They are built with great emphasis on modernity of
architecture, with many comforts for patients and
personnel; they are full of equipment that performs
amazing acts even if it is also costly and quickly
obsolete. They are staffed by a great variety of
people representing a multitude of professions and
skills, watched over by a board, directed by an administrator, accountable to several unions, and in
many areas financed wholly or in part by several levels of government. Their aim is an operation that is
efficient and which uses effectively all the technological advantages of the age. The challenge is to
retain the concern for the individual patient within
their complex institutional structure.

SOCIAL WORK
If the history of hospitals seems like an ill-
traced path, the history of social work is even more
so. Origins and motivations are ambiguous at least
until the nineteenth century.

Primitive tribes are usually thought of as ruth-
less to weakness but there would seem to be evidence
that even the most primitive nomadic tribes offered
assistance to individual members when they encountered
difficulties, though it might be only for reasons
of survival and self-preservation. The Old Testament
contains many references to assistance and commands

---

6. Will M. Carleton (1845-1912), Over the Hill to
the Poor House. Carleton was a prolific writer of
poetry and song. This rather long poem may be found
in a volume of The Best Loved Poems of the American
People.
7. Raymond P. Sloan, This Hospital Business of Ours
(New York, 1952), chap. II.

to people to help one another. Indeed, in the first
Book of Genesis, Verse 18, God makes it clear that
it was His intention that Eve was created to be a
"help meet" for Adam. Throughout the five books of
Moses there are definite and frequent admonitions
about helping others. The teaching of the New Testament expanded this concern greatly since it provided
a philosophy of charity based on the intrinsic meaning of love. For twenty centuries, the mixture of
beliefs that constitute the Judaeo-Christian ethic
has been a powerful social determinant that has
shaped the assumption of man's responsibility for his
fellow man, and this responsibility has been assumed
in many ways.

Until the time of the overthrow of the lords of
the manor, serfs expected and had a right to expect,
sustenance for all kinds of need. Those who left the
feudal land believed it was their right to beg and
the more fortunate felt that it was their privilege
to give them alms. Monasteries, with their hospital
adjuncts, were geared to serving people, as people
required their help.

However, as society became more complex sociological pressures caused changes. In the centuries preceding 1600, population increased, trade both domestic
and foreign became significant, the feudal system had
decayed, some travelling between other countries augmented and enlarged ideas, and economics and finance
had new roles to play. All these factors combined to
cause a shift away from earlier cultural patterns.
Populations began a move from rural to urban living,
towns and market places arose; with dislocation poverty, sickness and misery often resulted.

The famous Poor Law of 1601 was a result of an
attempt to control this situation and to give help.
For its time, it was an amazing social document, if
only in its concept that individuals could not always
provide for themselves and that governments, in this
instance the parish, must assume some responsibility.
However, there also was combined in it a basic philosophy that those in need should somehow be punished and
that punishment would be a deterrent in preventing
others from either requesting or needing help. Unfortunately, even though a broader and deeper concept
of human beings and their inherent rights developed,
the punitive and primitive thinking of the Poor Law
was slow to change. Its philosophy spread far and wide

and even to-day its residence clause is clutched
tightly in many pieces of welfare legislation. In
1834, England made minor modifications in the original
statute of 1601 but retained most of its punishing
attitudes. Quite naturally, because of a common British heritage, Canada and the United States incorporated in their social legislation theories and regulations from the English Poor Law; for example, families were automatically responsible for their relatives; the original place of residence must assume the
costs of financial assistance; that able-bodied individuals should work (whether there was work or not)
and therefore were not eligible for relief. But
developments in the social work and welfare fields
are not rooted only in the British tradition. Europ-
ean countries contributed their share. The concerned
citizens of Limoges, France, organized a community
chest as a means of obtaining relief moneys in the
fourteenth century. (Community chests, often called
United Appeal, became operative in North America in
the 1920's.) St. Vincent de Paul (1576-1660), a French-
man, exerted a great influence. Because of his love
and understanding of children, he built orphanages;
later, moved by a broader compassion, he built homes
for the aged and founded the Sisters of Charity, an
order of nuns, to care for the sick, the poor and the
young. Many other institutions could be cited. Their
functions are clearly contained in the names given to
these charitable organizations, e.g. xenodocia -- inns
for travellers and strangers; brephotropia -- found-
ling asylums; orphanotropia -- orphanages (note the
distinction between orphans and infants), and geron-
tokomia -- homes for the aged. But these efforts were
often sporadic and there were few attempts to continue
and develop these services in a vital way.

Over a period of historical time it can be seen
how pressures will gradually build up by which society
is modified, and a new concept of goals and new sets
of needs are recognized. The Industrial Revolution
provided a succession of changes, often abrupt and
violent, which could not fail to have important and
long-lasting effects on society. The dislocations of
this era brought about not only an affluent society
which has continued to this day, but also a gradually
more and more pressing need to find ways of dealing
with the many for whom the pace of advance was too
rapid or whom the benefits of the new technology did
not satisfactorily reach. Efforts were sporadic at

the beginning – an example would be when Austria and
France, in the early nineteenth century, began programs to assist workmen injured on the job or some old
age pensions. It is impossible here to do all these
efforts justice let alone record them, but their influence must be acknowledged in the development of
attitudes which considered provision for human needs
important.

Growth and proliferation of welfare schemes in
Europe and North America are striking phenomena of
the twentieth century. If any single catalyst is to
be defined that caused the mutation of cultural norms
in the twentieth century, it must be World War I, for
it was immediately following the Armistice that the
idea that this is one world began to germinate and
with it came a change in attitudes, philosophy and
behaviour which profoundly affected all kinds of human thinking and endeavour. [8] One area of this new
questioning was that of social well-being. Beginning
in 1929 and going on to 1948, built according to the
social architecture of Sir William Beveridge, a total
revision of the Elizabethan Poor Laws was enacted by
the National Assistance Bill. An attempt was made to
cover by legislation all human contingencies financed
both by government moneys and by individual contribu-
tions. The philosophy of assistance was affected and
now relief was considered a right not a privilege.
The people of Canada and the United States were also
undergoing great upheavals in their thinking about
human needs and their provisions for such needs. At
first, both countries enacted statutes on a piecemeal
basis and in a much less revolutionary manner. Industrial society has always known economic recessions,
but the great depression in the 1930's made it imper-
ative that these countries recognize governmental
responsibilities in these areas of human well-being.
Since then, countless welfare programs, costing bil-
lions of tax dollars, have become an integral part
of the North American culture. In the formulation and
application of all these, social work philosophy has

---

8. For a detailed review of this period The Proud
Tower: A Portrait of the World before the War, 1890-
1914 by Barbara W. Tuchman (New York, 1966), is
well worth reading.

been influential and social workers have helped shape
their structure. It was after all from the private
agencies that first-hand knowledge came of what was
happening to people. Schooled and matured in the
voluntary or private agencies and philanthropies for
over a hundred years, social workers were particularly qualified to act not only as the yeast but the
dough itself in these programs.

The enactment and utilization of government sponsored programs in the welfare field belong to the
recent past. Almost a hundred years before this development numerous individuals were joining together to
give themselves and their worldly goods to help the
unfortunate. Social work did, indeed, begin with the
volunteer and the Lady Bountiful and infinite credit
must be given to these men and women for their vision
and understanding of the fact that real and constructive help cannot be given on a part-time do-good basis.
Acting from motives of charity, love of neighbour,
love of God, pity and compassion, organizations soon
to be called agencies were founded, that help might
be provided more realistically and more constructively so that the money available would be spent more
wisely.

Human beings of magnificent personality who ac-
complish much for humanity often seem to have a
strongly mystical and impassioned quality. The individuals of the nineteenth century who were the begin-
ners in the field of social work manifested this in
great measure. Among them were Octavia Hill (1838-
1912), Elizabeth Fry (1780-1845), Canon Samuel
Barnett (1844-1913), and Mary Richmond (1861-1928).
Perhaps to select these four is unfair: there are
hundreds of others who gave their lives to easing the
pain of suffering humanity. The Encyclopedia of
Social Work published in 1965 by the National Association of Social Workers contains brief biographies
of some of them.

It is today generally recognized that the
first organized social agency was the Charity Organization Society of London, known affectionately for
nearly 100 years as the C.O.S., but first bearing the
awesome title, The Society for Organizing Charitable
Relief and Repressing Mendicity. It was founded in
1869 and its three purposes were clearly stated:
(1) the organizing of relief giving; (2) the control
of mendicants; (3) improvement of the poor. The C.O.S.
built its philosophy and program on charitable endea-

vours that preceded it, such as church-based visitors
and local relief-giving societies. Its members were
dedicated to uplifting the deprived, saving the fallen
and protecting the abused, as well as the abolition
of drunkenness,gambling and other vices. At first,
the staff were volunteers but within two years it was
recognized that this method of staffing was not adequate to fulfil the aims of the Society and the necessity of having full-time paid workers was recognized. Usually, these were ladies of considerable refinement and gentility and one cannot but sympathize
with them because of the shocks, rebuffs and antago-
nism that must have been their lot. Undoubtedly, the
reaction of many of their friends and relatives was
scorching and their sensitivities must have often
been outraged and trampled as they went among the
poor and the downtrodden in East London and in the
dock areas. But they persevered and a C.O.S. movement grew and spread not only in the British Isles
but in North America. In 1877, Buffalo, N.Y., established one of the first such agencies. Philadelphia,
New York, Boston, Baltimore, Montreal and Toronto
followed soon and from these infant organizations developed the whole broad range of family agencies now
functioning in cities and towns throughout the world.
These agencies are known by mutations of the original
name: Family Welfare Association, Family Service Bu-
reau, or Family Service Association. Their names denote their purpose: to give service to families; they
are the corner-stone of all community resources because without a good family agency, other agencies
with a more specialized function cannot operate adequately.
      These more specialized concerns gave rise to
organizations or societies that had as their aim care
of children, the aged, the prisoners, the mentally
ill and the physically sick. Settlement houses were
established in slum neighbourhoods in which workers
lived in order to be accessible to the people who
needed them. These houses, many founded as the result
of a religious conviction, became potent forces under
the direction of inspired leadership. The **first**,
Toynbee Hall, was opened Christmas Eve, 1884, in White-
chapel, by Canon Barnett. The stories of Henry St.
Settlement on New York's Lower East Side and Hull
House in Chicago of the early 1900's are fascinating

documentaries. Lillian Wald (1867-1940) and Jane
Addams (1860-1935) were the crusaders. The YM and
YWCA, and later the YM and WHA, with roots in religious convictions, were also instruments of social
help. Children's institutions and orphanages and
later, just after 1900, Children's Aid Societies were
founded not only to give material help but protection
to children. Medical social work began in 1895 and
psychiatric in 1913.

These many endeavours required staff and before
long that staff was asking for training. Education
for social work was the dream of one of the most courageous, realistic yet visionary, women in the history of social work, Mary Richmond (1861-1929). And
it was most fitting that in 1898, under the aegis of
the New York C.O.S., it was she who taught the first
class of social workers to undertake formal learning
at the summer school of Philanthropic Workers. Social
work had lost much of its Lady Bountiful tradition
and already had "a philosophy which embodied many of
the principles of modern casework and a technique
which could be transmitted by education and training
from one generation of social workers to the next."[9]

Miss Richmond worked in Baltimore, Philadelphia
and New York, and gave to the profession such books
as What is Social Casework, Social Diagnosis, and
The Long View, as well as many articles. It was she
who admonished social workers, long before Freudian
theory became popular, to look to the underlying
meaning of behaviour.

Social work exists in and reflects back society
at any given point in time. In considering its history then, it is not strange to find that its growth,
development and refinement have many facets. In the
beginning, it was concerned with those whom society
considered unfortunate and with the social problems
of poverty and disease, and its activities were centered around the giving of material goods. During
the hungry thirties, social workers came to realize
with startling clarity that their efforts would be
effective only if governments got fully in step with
the realities of modern economic and industrial life,
and if they themselves learned more about the causes

---

9. Kathleen Woodroofe, From Charity to Social Work,
p. 54.

and effects of human behaviour. Doctors such as Freud and his disciples Jung and Adler, William Alanson White and Harry Stack Sullivan were beginning to make an impression on world thought. The cataclysm of World War II shook people into a recognition that human beings acted dynamically. Because the leaders and teachers of social work in the 30's and 40's were closely linked with such organizations as universities and hospitals, it is not strange that they, if only by osmosis, absorbed psychoanalytical theory from the psychiatrists and psychoanalysts of all schools of thought and different doctrines, nor is it strange that the social work profession took up psychiatric knowledge, adjusting its skills and techniques and perhaps often straining thereby some of the important elements of its role and function. Inevitably, confusion ensued and in the late fifties emphasis began to be placed again on the social in social work.

Social workers then, are moulded by society and reflect society in their work. Consequently, it is not surprising to find that in the 1950's there was a noticeable shift in the philosophy of social workers and in agency programs. With the assumption of relief giving in large part by governmental agencies, social workers voluntarily or at times unconsciously responded to subtle societal pressures, withdrew to the less specific service of social work treatment and dealt mainly with a middle class clientele. The agency and social work rationalized this by the attitude that the relief-giving source (government agency) should also give a full service including that of social work treatment. There was, of course, in these years the upward mobility of the wage earner class into a new and enlarged stratum of the middle class. However, in the middle sixties, there has been a rediscovery of the culture of poverty and of the needs of the poor. Social work literature, as reflected in The Journal of Social Work, published by the National Association of Social Workers, Social Case Work, published by the Family Service Association of America, The Social Worker, published by the Canadian Association of Social Workers, are excellent source material on this topic. However, the basic premise of social work has survived - the worth of the human being as an individual made up of physical, social, emotional and spiritual parts. And it is with this humanistic value orientation that social work must function.

MEDICAL SOCIAL WORK

Hippocrates (450-345 B.C.), so many centuries ago, knew that illness could not be treated apart from the patient and his family. He wrote: "It is necessary for the physician to provide not only needed treatment but to provide for the sick man himself and for those beside him, and to provide for his <u>outside affairs</u>" (italics mine).

Perhaps the early hospitals, being so close in time and place to Hippocrates, fulfilled this mandate as did those first established under the auspices of the monasteries. However, the pious belief that sickness was God's punishment for sin did much to deter intervention on behalf of the sufferer and held back the development of social work in health settings. Later, the microscope and the telescope both narrowed and enlarged knowledge and when medicine grew more and more scientific, the part of the patient that defied material classification came to be ignored. Indeed, medical social work had to await the evolution of a philosophy concerning the value of man. It was in the latter half of the nineteenth century that, once again, patients became bodies and souls with the word soul meaning everything other than physical characteristics. However, a good idea never really dies; sometimes, it only lies dormant for centuries to be revived as something new; in this context the concern for the social being of the patient which was to be given over to the care of the almoners at the end of the nineteenth century.

The word almoner is an interesting one and apparently is a derivative of the word eleemosynarius (L eleemosyna -- alms); the person so called was the dispenser of alms for the monasteries. The first connotation of social worker was the giver of charity or alms. This concept carried over to the hospital setting and the first social workers in hospitals were called almoners. In America, social workers in hospitals were first called hospital social workers, and later, medical social workers. [10] But apparently long before the first almoner, some hospitals had a Samaritan Society that provided a fund from which

---

10. Mary A. Stites, <u>History of the American Association of Medical Social Workers</u> (American Association of Medical Social Workers, 1955), pp. 1-7.

material assistance was given to discharged patients, particularly to those who needed money to pay for transportation home. Evans and Howard relate a touching story taken from Gray's History of English Philanthropy about a "cripple with a new pair of crutches and a shilling," [11] trying to get himself home to Gloucestershire. Somebody saw and understood the problem of transportation and so, in 1791, Samaritan Societies were formed to care for such need. Transportation of patients is obviously not a problem of the twentieth century, and many medical social workers have reason to feel that it has been growing like a snowball since 1791.

The beginning of medical social work is usually dated January 1, 1895, in England, but there is a record of home visiting being done under the aegis of the Children's Hospital in San Francisco in 1886, and the New York Babies Hospital in 1894. Several other hospitals in Boston and New York also developed a home visitors program.[12] The history of these efforts is unfortunately vague but the concern felt by the hospital and the medical staff for helpless human beings is obvious. It would appear that previously,in the early 1870's, in England, doctors were beginning to manifest uneasiness about the great mass of London's poor. Committees were formed and discussion centered around the worthiness of free patients and whether or not a fee for out-patient treatment should be charged, and if so, how much. Also there was anxiety about patients and their families who might be in need of financial assistance. The talk in committees went on from 1872 until Charles Loch, secretary of the C.O.S., became involved. [13]

Loch (later Sir Charles Loch) must have been a man of rare sensibilities. During his student days at Oxford, he joined the Fabian Society because he believed that their philosophy offered a framework

11. Delbert Evans and I.G. Redmont Howard, The Romance of the British Voluntary Hospital Movement (London, 1930), p. 241.

12. Ida Canon, On the Social Frontiers of Medicine (Howard University Press, 1952, chaps. 2 and 3.)

13. Ibid., pp. 12-13.

within which society could grow and refine its institutions. A biography of Sir Charles Loch has not
been written, but Kathleen Woodroofe in her book
From Charity to Social Work, working from source
material, has assembled quotations from his writings
that reveal his remarkable intensity of soul and
spirit of charity. She quotes him as saying that he
had "a vague regret that the lives of others judged
by his own were sunless and sad." [14] Moved by this
feeling he devoted his life, his intellect and his
emotions to others including the sick poor. As a result of his efforts, a member of his staff, Miss
Mary Stewart, was lent to the Royal Free Hospital
for three months and so became the first almoner.
Her responsibilities were outlined clearly; she was
charged with: (1) preventing abuse of the hospital
by persons able to pay for medical treatment, (2) re-
ferring patients already in receipt of parish relief
and such as are destitute to the Poor Law authorities, (3) recommending suitable persons to join Pro-
vident Dispensaries. [15] Being the kind of man he was,
it is not unlikely that Loch's concern was less about
patients cheating the hospital but more about patients themselves. They were admitted sick and worn,
kept in hospital until they were made well, and sent
home to the same surroundings and under the same circumstances that had made them sick in the first place
only to return to clinic in a few weeks time again
ill and debilitated.

   Although Miss Stewart's tenure expired in three
months and the hospital refused to allocate the necessary funds to re-employ her, her work had made so
great an impact that the doctors and the hospital
were forced to consider patient care in a broader
perspective and, after further negotiations, Miss
Stewart returned to the hospital staff. Miss Stewart
had ably demonstrated the value both to the patient
and the hospital, of social treatment for problems
that caused illness and prevented patients from
getting well. She realized quickly the futility of
prescribing milk for children when there was no bread

---

14. Kathleen Woodroofe, From Charity to Social Work,
p. 22.

15. Ida Cannon, On the Social Frontiers of Medicine,
p. 17.

for anyone or vacation for a **wife w**hose husband went on his weekly drunk on Saturday night and beat her up on Sunday morning. Her work became known and other hospitals employed their own almoners, one of the most illustrious being Miss Anne E. Cummins of St. Thomas Hospital. And so, the hospital almoner movement was born and social work in the hospital organization had begun.

Dr. Richard Cabot introduced it to North America. Everything that is known about Dr. Cabot bears witness to his great and deep humanity, his concern for people, his appreciation of the human being and his unflagging devotion to the sick. It was inevitable that in 1905, when he returned to Boston and the Massachusetts General Hospital after a period of studies in London, he should establish what was the first structured social service department in a hospital on the North American Continent. Although he met with great opposition from many hospitals and a multitude of doctors, such outstanding individuals in the field of medicine as Sir William Osler, then at Oxford, Dr. T.S. Armstrong of Bellevue Hospital and Dr. Daniel Gilman of Johns Hopkins Hospital supported and encouraged him.

It is often difficult to know in retrospect all the diverse societal forces that are interacting at a given point in time and combine to produce a movement, a discovery or, indeed, a personality. But apparently, the first decade of the twentieth century was a point in time when people began to care again about the poor and the sick, and hospitals, particularly in the larger cities in the United States and in Montreal, Quebec, established social service departments as instruments of help. In 1929, The American College of Physicians and Surgeons, in their Report on Hospital Standardization, recognized "the valuable assistance in diagnosis and treatment" of social work though the recognition was largely on paper at first. Cities in Canada, outside the province of Quebec, were much slower to develop this service, but by the 1960's awareness of the contribution of social work in the treatment of the sick is growing and social work in medical settings is more widely accepted. But the growth has been slow. In 1960, the American Hospital Association conjointly with the National Association of Social Workers published Essentials

of a Social Service Department in Hospitals and Related Institutions. 16
     Social workers learned long ago that social
problems seek not only the poor and medical social
workers have long been convinced of the value of
their help to the sick, not just to the poor sick,
but the sick. To quote Dr. J.H. Means: "Medical
Social Service is not only for the poor alone, but
for any patient in whose case a social problem exists.
Medical Social Service is just what its name implies.
It is a service, not a charity. Its service embraces
a skill which enables the effective carrying out in
our complex society of the medical treatment that the
doctor of medicine prescribes."17 The social problems
that are created or accentuated by illness require
treatment if the patient is to return to a maximal
level of health in its comprehensive sense. Far too
frequently, individuals struggle ineptly and unsatis-
factorily with a problem in their social environment
that causes illness and often it is only when they
become physically ill that they are free to understand
and accept their need for help and so permit themselves to be helped by social work skills and techniques.

SUMMARY

     Social work is a profession whose body of know-
ledge, skills and techniques are and may be learned
for the sole purpose of helping human beings in social difficulties whether the malfunction occurs
because of interpersonal dysfunction or environmental
stress. It is based on a firm belief in the value of
the individual human being, and the aim of assisting
him to achieve a mode of living that produces some
satisfaction for himself and helps him make a positive
contribution to society. Its primary focus is the
social functioning of the individual. Medical social
work is social work practised in or under the auspices of an organization or institution whose primary

16. Essentials ofaSocial Service Department in Hospitals and Related Institutions (American Hospital
Association, 840 North Lake Shore Dr.,Chicago, Ill.,
1961).
17. Ida Cannon, On the Social Frontiers of Medicine,
p. 18.

objective is treatment of any kind of illness.

The histories, herein so crudely related, of hospitals and social work are inextricably bound. Evans and Howard summarize: "The central idea of the earliest attempts at a hospital system was charity rather than science, care rather than cure, religion rather than medicine." 18 It is possible in our modern hospitals to-day to have both charity _and_ science, care _and_ cure, religion _and_ medicine.

---

18. Evans and Howard, _British Voluntary Hospital Movement_, p. 13.

CHAPTER III

A FRAME FOR MEDICAL SOCIAL WORK

"It is clear that social work is concerned
with both the person (or group) and the
social environment, that is, the person in
the situation. This implies a biophysio-
social perspective which cuts across the
boundaries of knowledge and of the disciplines as currently defined." 1

An understanding of the role of medical social work
has to be based on a comprehension of the nature and
aims of social work itself since medical social work
is social work practised in a health setting whether
it be a general or specialized hospital, health department or a community clinic. The phrase social work
in health settings is too cumbersome for daily use,
so it is usually called medical social work. At the
present time there is a trend, particularly in the
United States, to use the descriptive phrase "clin-
ical social work." Also, social work itself may be
a term needing definition: confusion can be created
if it is not distinguished from the all-inclusive
term social welfare. Social welfare, simply stated,
means programs and legislation established or enacted
by any level of government for the social well-being
of its people. The purpose of this chapter is to
state a few basic facts about the profession of social work. It is not meant to be all embracing.

SOCIAL WORK
   A definition of social work, equally simply
stated, presents it as a profession within the framework of which help is given to individuals or groups

---

1. Harry L. Lurie, Encyclopedia of Social Work
(published by National Association of Social Workers,
New York, N.Y. 1965), p. 759

who are experiencing social dysfunction. Of course,
like any definition,this one is inadequate to de-
scribe the practice of social work or to suggest the
various activities which are necessary to make
practice viable and effective. It is comparable to
defining the practice of medicine as the art of healing. Either statement requires expansion.

Consideration of the hallmarks of a profession
will assist in giving substance to our definition.
A profession is characterized by: (1) its own body
of knowledge that may be learned; (2) its own methodology and techniques; (3) its own code of ethics;
(4) use of these in service to human beings. Social
work has its own body of knowledge, even though,
like every other profession, it has incorporated
ideas and facts from many sources; also, like every
other profession, it has adjusted them to a form
suitable for its own use. It has its own methodology,
applied by consciously learned techniques that are
specific to social work practice. It has its own code
of ethics constantly under scrutiny by the professional associations. Its goal is to facilitate the
achievement of satisfactory social functioning of
individuals or groups.

The practice of social work within a professional frame of reference is, then, recognized by "a
constellation of value, purpose, sanction, knowledge
and method." [2] It is a unique arrangement and application of these elements that distinguish social work
from other professions. In discussing the nature of
social work, Boehm emphasizes its essential values:
"the values [listed here] are thought to be compatible
with those held in the culture of the United States
and Canada. They express more specifically such widely held values of democratic society as the worth of
the individual, the inherent dignity of the human
person, society's responsibility for individual welfare and the individual's responsibility for contributing to the common good." [3]

---

2. Harriet M. Bartlett, "Toward Clarification and
Improvement of Social Work Practice" (Journal of
Social Work, Vol. 3, No. 2, April, 1958), p. 5.

3. Werner Boehm, "The Nature of Social Work" (Journal
of Social Work, Vol. 3, No. 2, April, 1958), p. 11.

The aims of social work are two: (1) to help an individual live in such a way that his life pattern is satisfying to him, and (2) to help him be a contributing member of the community. The word "contributing" may have a simple connotation as well as a more complex one: it does not need to imply a momentous act of science or a great work of art. An aged person, helped live out the days of his years at peace with himself and his surroundings, is making contribution enough. The emphasis of social work on a belief in the worth of every individual is important and it carries with it an aim to give persons at least an opportunity for help in adjusting to stress. In the early twenties Mary Richmond emphasized the importance of recognizing the reality of the personality, and some fifteen years later, Gordon Hamilton emphasized the strength life's experiences can have for the individual. Very frequently the human organism, subjected to the stress of these realities, is unable to cope with them, not necessarily because of any inherent deficiency in him but because of the power of the reality itself. Social work, however, is not absolved from further responsibility for humanity by this concentration on an individual; it must concern itself also with society and its value systems and with how it assumes its responsibility for the individual. Consequently, in order to keep faith with its professional orientation, social work must demand of its practitioners that they learn and develop competence in understanding the meaning of human behaviour within the social context, and how to help the individual whose behaviour has become abnormal or unsatisfying to him.

Obviously, education for the professional practice of social work is essential. Full professional qualification requires a long and expensive period of study. It proceeds from a Bachelor of Arts degree or its equivalent and then satisfactory meeting of the requirements of a two-year curriculum in an accredited school of social work. (The accrediting body for Canada and the United States is the Council on Social Work Education, 345 E-46th St., New York 17, N.Y.). It is the body of professional knowledge that must be learned, the skills and techniques that must be acquired, and the philosophy of social work that must be absorbed which make this long training

necessary. Moreover, admission to a school of social
work has to be based not only on a Bachelor of Arts
degree but also on a personality potentially adapt-
able to giving service to people in trouble. An applicant will be screened, before he is accepted, in
a pre-admission interview by the school of social
work. The two long and arduous years of study and
supervised practice combine both classroom study and
field work placement, at the end of which the student
is just beginning to learn to use himself and his
knowledge. The social worker thus endeavours to syn-
thesize elements of value, knowledge, method and art
which are all to be consciously learned and then used
specifically in social work treatment.

Treatment of social problems is given by one or
a combination of three methods: casework, group work
and community organization. Students are required to
have an understanding of all three methods, but major
in one, and they need to be familiar with social research and administration. Completion of this study
gives admission to two professional associations:
The National Association of Social Workers in the
United States and The Canadian Association of Social
Workers in Canada, each with district, state or provincial organizations. In Canada, most provincial
associations are autonomous but have representation
in the national organization. Eligibility for membership is determined basically by the achievement of
the Master's Degree. However, the Canadian Association of Social Workers has an ongoing committee on
membership whose charge it is to review the qualifications for membership of workers from countries who
do not have the same educational background as that
obtained in North American Schools of Social Work.
At the same time it is examining the professional
credentials of graduates in the welfare courses given
by the Technical Colleges.

In recent years, the demands for staff by social
and welfare agencies have exceeded by thousands the
number of those with Master's degrees who have been
graduated from Schools of Social Work, or indeed,
that can be educated in such schools. Consequently,
the profession has had to take a careful look at
other ways of preparing people at different levels
of education to do different levels of jobs in social
and welfare organizations. Some universities and
colleges are offering optional courses in their li-

beral arts programs, and the profession hopes that
these will give students both the knowledge and the
encouragement that will enable them to undertake
professional education. Some universities are offering an undergraduate course in social work. The University of Windsor, Windsor, Ontario, started such a
course in September, 1966. Laurentian University in
Sudbury, Ontario, offered a similar one in 1967 and
McMaster University in Hamilton, Ontario, expects to
begin its undergraduate course in social work in
September, 1968. Also, technical institutes in Van-
couver, Brandon, Toronto, Montreal and Halifax have
already graduated social work assistants. The same
kind of technical social work education is included
in community colleges located in Brampton, Hamilton,
St. Catharines, Scarborough and North York. Undoubtedly, these particular kinds of educational opportunities will increase and the graduates will be employed
for specific tasks defined in accordance with their
skills and performed under professional supervision.
      Social work is practised in many fields and with-
in many organizational structures. The largest number
of workers are in primary agencies such as family
agencies, child care agencies, group or recreational
agencies, and in organizations established to serve
a specific purpose: senior citizens, a membership
group, a special problem (e.g., Old Age Clubs, Big
Brothers, and Social Planning Councils). However, an
increasing number of social workers are employed in
secondary settings such as institutions, governmental
departments serving a wide range of programs, courts,
clinics, and hospitals of all kinds. It must be noted
that the basic or generic training, i.e. casework,
group work, or community organization remains constant, but their application and emphasis change with
the setting and the focus of the organization in
which they are practised.

MEDICAL SOCIAL WORK
      Illness is a social event that affects not only
the ill person, but also his family and may cause
disruption in all aspects of their living. Illness
is inexorable in its choice and plays no favourites;
poor and rich alike are its victims. Indisputably,
the dislocation caused by sickness and hospitalization varies in degree, according to the person,

without reference to the diagnosis or severity of the disease or the economic status of the patient. "She doesn't need a social worker, her husband is loaded," is sometimes heard, but a severe dysfunction may thereby be dismissed: money may be the very reason she does need a social worker.

The social implications of illness beyond its physical effects are receiving more and more attention in recent years. Both the medical and the nursing professions are producing a flood of books and articles on the subject of total care including in their educational approach an enlargement of knowledge and understanding of the human and personal needs and reactions of patients. Their own emphasis remains, of course, on the knowledge and techniques pertinent to their own professions. The social worker in the hospital organization represents the discipline whose professional focus is the social functioning of the patient and his family.

It has long been known that social stress can make an individual sick, and longer recognized that sickness can and does cause fear, depression, a breakdown in family and other relationships, economic hardship because of loss or lowering of income or changes in personal and family standards of living. For all or any of these conditions the result may be broken homes and broken lives. There are other social dysfunctions too, some of which are becoming more urgent with every year of scientific change and technological progress, such as the need for post-discharge care, adjustment of the pattern of living of the nuclear family and provision and use of medical services after hospitalization. The knowledge, skills and techniques of social work are more and more being recognized as an essential part of the over-all treatment of illness and are increasingly provided by hospitals for their patients.

SUMMARY
Social work is a profession whose body of knowledge, skills and techniques are learned for the purpose of helping human beings in social difficulties whether the malfunction occurs because of interpersonal dysfunction or environmental stress. It is based on a firm belief in the value of the individual

human being, and in his potential to achieve a mode
of living that produces some satisfaction for himself
and helps him make a positive contribution to society.
It is a profession whose primary focus is the social
functioning of the individual. Medical social work
is social work practised in or under the auspices of
an organization or institution whose primary objective is treatment of any kind of illness.

CHAPTER IV

ATTITUDES

> "The open door, the open mind, the
> willingness to think things through
> all over again no matter how many
> times, those, I suppose, are the things
> that keep organizations as well as
> people young." 1

In chapters II and III an effort was made by consideration of historical trends to provide a wide
screen on which social work in the hospital organization was depicted as in a three-dimensional picture.
We now turn to yet another presentation of context,
and to the attitudes which may be associated with
the hospital itself. We shall then move on to a
discussion of the present role and function of social
work in the hospital.

The word hospital may have different meanings.
Its Latin derivation is from a combination of "hos-
pes," both host and guest, and "hospitium," a place
where a guest was received. In essence, "hospital"
suggests three elements: host, guest, and place,
with inter-dependency among them implied. The modern
hospital represents an accumulation of custom and
tradition out of the experience of sixteen hundred
years, and has been shaped and re-shaped by the ebb
and flow of human knowledge and expectation. At
various times the hospital has been looked upon in
a variety of ways: as a refuge, even as a charnel-
house in unhappy periods of its history, a centre
for developing scientific knowledge, and a place for
treatment of the sick and injured. More recently,
the last two have had chief stress. Similarly, at
times the organization of a hospital has shown shifts
of emphasis from the religious order, to the board,
and, with the advent of sepsis and medical education,

---

1. Mary Richmond, The Long View (New York: Russell
Sage Foundation 1930), p. 277.

to the doctor. For at least the last two generations,
the doctor particularly has perceived the hospital to
be a setting where he has had broad authority and
power, a position that is, indeed, inherent in his
special knowledge of and responsibility for life and
death. In the last few decades the rising operating
costs, the establishment of health and hospital insurance plans and the growth in population, have
brought the community into a closer connection with
hospitals. It makes this connection through the board
of directors. These boards have assumed interest in
and responsibility for the actual policies and procedures of hospital operations. The judgment by which
these boards function in any individual situation
reflects, of course, their understanding of what is
inherent in their responsibility and their attitudes
to other positions of authority. There is yet another
element to-day in the hospital world. The development
of hospital administration as a profession requiring
distinct skills and knowledge has occurred since W.W.
II; hospital administration responsibilities have
thus been given to non-medical persons who are educated for their particular role. The administrator,
who has inevitably acquired attitudes consistent with
his own profession, finds himself between the board
and the community on one hand and the medical and
paramedical professions on the other. Strains im-
plicit in these juxtapositions may well come to the
fore when the budget is prepared or when new policies
that affect both patients and staff must be adapted.

Yet another attitude to be taken into any account
of the hospital context is that of patients. Undoubtedly, there are a large number of patients and their
families who understand the value of modern hospital
care and welcome admission. But there are many whose
attitudes prevent them from accepting hospitalization
or from deriving full benefit from it. Every hospitalized patient knows an element of conscious or unconscious fear. Dr. Perry Pepper expressed this when
he wrote "fear is every doctor's enemy and every
patient's bed-fellow. Fear multiplies the social
worker's problems, tests the nurse's tact and patience
and lessens the doctor's chance to save." 2

2. D.H.P. Pepper, M.D. "The Patient's Fears,"Journal
of Nervous Diseases, Vol. 82, 1935, p. 369.

Such fears are lively survivors of the not-so-distant
time when "going to hospital" meant that both the
doctor and the family, not to mention the patient,
knew that death was immediate. Other well-known negative reactions on the part of patients include that
against "being used for experiments" and being "practised on by students." An elderly patient, to take
another example, felt that his very identity was
effaced in hospital and refused further admission
because "they took away my pants and made me wear
their things" (hospital gowns). These emotional reactions are found to-day in both rural and urban
populations. Certainly the impersonality of the large
modern hospital has an effect upon the life of the
patient in it, as Stephen Becker has described. [3]

The modern hospital, staffed by qualified personnel from many professional disciplines using a
variety of work skills and administered professionally, is indeed a community resource. Society uses
it as one of its instruments to promote physical,
social, emotional, and mental health, and it is in
this context that hospitals have to be considered.
Modern hospitals normally subscribe to two funda-
mental principles determining and governing their
role and function in society. First, they conceive
of themselves as an instrument shaped and used by
society to give total care to the sick. Secondly,
taking this as their mandate, they must provide and
make available the many different and special resources, both in personnel and equipment, necessary
to give total care. The public has certainly had an
influence here. The various media of communication
in the modern world have provided it with a sophisti-
cation in its knowledge of medical science, as well
as a need for a range of doctors representing a
wide spectrum of medical specialities and the provision of ever increasing facilities for care in the
hospital. It has also come to expect a much higher
level of arrangements for physical comfort. To-day
there are more hospitals, with more facilities,
housing more pieces of equipment, with larger budgets
and engaged in an eternal struggle for personnel than

---

3. Stephen Becker, "On Being a Patient," Atlantic
Monthly, July, 1966, pp. 45-101.

ever before in recorded time. [4]

Within this context of the modern hospital --
comprised of boards of directors, medical personnel
(doctors and nurses and the great variety of those
associated with them), administrative staff, and patients --the social worker must find her place. In
addition to developing an understanding of the professional role her particular training fits her to
fill within this complicated context -- a point which
has been introduced in the preceding chapter and will
be elaborated in those that follow -- she must also
find her way among the attitudes to her and her work
which she may encounter. As has been noted previously,
it can occur that among these attitudes is one of
question whether social work does indeed have a function in the hospital setting, and the question can
sometimes be put sharply. The reason for such questioning may be as simple as dissatisfaction with the
performance of a social worker, to which the reply
is, of course, that as in any group, there may be
individuals who are not sufficiently proficient in
their skills or whose understanding of their role is
not adequate. But the reasons may be more complex,
including often an element of misinformation. A brief
discussion of them here may be helpful.

Information about social work itself and about
hospitals can be supplied from the literature that
continues to increase on these subjects. Social
agencies, professional organizations, hospitals, and
provincial hospital organizations all have relevant
informational material, free upon request. More leadership can, however, still be given by hospital organizations and the social work profession by way of
supporting their members and presenting their role to
the community.

Other attitudes of questioning may arise from
more hidden sources. It may be that a community as
represented by its board and its political leaders
maintains a comfortable conviction that "what was good
for our forefathers is good enough for us"; "We have
never done that" gives voice to this attitude. An
element of this conviction may also be the idea that

---

4. "The Trouble with Hospitals," Atlantic Monthly,
July 1966, pp. 88-123.

a person needing social help is simply someone who
lacks the stamina and thrift that other members of
the community display, and that this should be dis-
couraged. Patient presentation of today's needs,
which are often not those of yesterday, is necessary
in answer to this attitude.

Every community has individuals within it who
have an important influence on community projects
for reasons of financial or inherited prestige. They
may well have personal interests in particular
charitable or welfare or medical projects or organizations, which for this reason receive special financial aid or public notice. Professional people working in the community may often find this local fact
of life a cause of concern when it interferes with
what they consider urgent needs for a family agency
or a recreational centre, or the development of social service in the hospital setting. Such situations are never easy ones in which to work, but their
existence has to be recognized.

All of us are familiar with the notion of vested
interests. The world of welfare is no stranger to
these. Volunteers, for instance, who have had a long
and honourable tradition of service in the welfare
field, may question, even actively resent, the establishment of a social service department in a hospital,
feeling that their own program will decline in importance. Doctors working in hospitals are today finding
that technological advances (including the computer)
and new administrative methods are having an effect
on their position of authority and complicating the
traditional physician - patient relationship which
their profession has so stressed. Emergence of a
social service unit in their midst may at times be
seen by them as a possible further encroachment, or
may be, depending on the nature of their medical
education, imperfectly understood as an adjunct to
medical treatment. Such stresses within the hospital
itself (others could be mentioned) are valuable for
social service workers to be aware of and to make
allowance for, while at the same time maintaining
in themselves and encouraging in others confidence
in their own role.

Faint-heartedness about the establishment or
expansion of social service departments may occur
because of the pressure for funds in all health

services. Pressure is undeniable, but in these days
when government support of such services will certainly increase, it can sometimes be a pretext hiding
reactions such as those described above. Similarly
the obvious scarcity of trained personnel poses a
difficulty; again, it could be made a pretext. To-
day efforts (described in an earlier chapter) are
being made to increase and diversify training programs; moreover, the adequacy of salary, office
arrangements, and personnel policies are important
in attracting staff (a subject to be discussed
further in Chapter VI).

SUMMARY
        The strength of the attitudes of a community at
large and the attitudes within a hospital community
itself have an important effect on the place of social work in a hospital organization. However, a hospital with a social service department staffed by
professionally trained workers functioning within
the profession of social work and the hospital organization, is best able to fulfil its obligation to
give total care to its patients. Presentation of this
role requires education of relevant opinion and understanding of the tensions outlined in this chapter.

CHAPTER V

ROLE AND FUNCTION

"Man has four basic requirements --
philosophical adjustment, psychological
tolerance, sociological security, and
religious integration." [1]

The words role and function are often confused and
are even sometimes used interchangeably; an indus-
trious student in a graduate course once told a
professor that in one year he had counted 54 different meanings for the word role. A definition of
these terms within the particular frame of reference
of this book seems essential for clarity. As used
here, role is meant to indicate part or place.
Function is used to refer to the kind of action or
activity proper to a person or institution which is
necessary to fulfil its role; hence it refers to job
activity. (These definitions are substantiated by
the American College Dictionary, published by Random
House, New York, 1963.) It is obvious that a person
or institution may have one or several roles each
demanding a different function. For example: a man
may be a son to his parents, a husband to his wife,
a father to his children, and an employer to his
workers. Each of these parts or roles requires from
him different functions or activities. Similarly,
the role of the court in society is to adjudicate in
legal cases and to dispense justice. The functions
that are essential to this role are many: appointment
of judges, recognition of lawyers, provision of law
libraries and sundry personnel. It must be remembered
that expectations for a particular role or function
change not only with the changing times, but at the
same point in time may also vary from one community
to another.

---

1. Joshua Loth Liebman, Hope for Man (New York:
Simon and Schuster 1966), p. 149

ROLE OF THE SOCIAL SERVICE DEPARTMENT

The role of the social service department is to provide an administrative unit in the hospital organization within which and from which social workers are enabled to carry out their professional duties in cooperation with other personnel. The place of the social service department in the organizational structure thus enables planning, coordination and supervision of social work and social workers in the hospital.

FUNCTIONS OF THE SOCIAL SERVICE DEPARTMENT

The functions or job activities necessary for the exercise of the department's role are varied. They have to be determined within both the framework of the social work profession and the hospital organizational structure by the director of the department in collaboration with and with the support of the hospital administrator. These functions include:

1. Administration of all matters concerning social work itself and those related to the activities of the social workers.
2. Formulation of a social work program for the hospital.
3. Recruitment and supervision of social work staff.
4. Teaching and providing information about the social aspects of illness.
5. Liaison with community programs and projects related to health and welfare.
6. Research in social aspects of illness.

THE ROLE OF THE SOCIAL WORKER

The role of the social worker is to provide trained service in matters related to the social functioning of the patient. This role becomes possible by virtue of specific professional training and experience and is maintained with the support of the social service department as defined above. This statement should not be taken to imply that every patient in a hospital requires the attention of a social worker, or that only a social worker is able to help a patient with non-medical problems. It does affirm that the social worker is normally the person

on the treatment team who is able to speak with particular authority about the handling of social problems and whose authority in this area is substantiated by professional knowledge, methodology, and experience. An earlier chapter has discussed the sometimes difficult context in which this role is performed. It is both prudent and necessary to keep the
definition in mind and to maintain it with conviction
as well as tact. In a paper given at an institute of
the Social Work Section of the Ontario Hospital Association, April 1966, Leona Grossman referred to the
anxieties social workers may have in relation to medical authority and advised that if these were "to
blur our [social workers'] perspectives in assuming
our professional responsibility, we capitulate our
professional commitment in helping people." She went
on to say: "we [social workers] can very logically
insist on the basis of what we have come to know
about the sick role, that a medical disposition which
does not link with a social disposition is not going
to work out." [2]

THE FUNCTION OF THE SOCIAL WORKER
     The functions or job activities of the hospital
social worker are performed in many ways but always
within the frame of reference of her hospital and
within her social work competence. The basic job may
be described by means of three relationships: (1)
with the patient; (2) within the hospital; (3) outside the hospital.
     1. With the patient.
     (a) direct social work treatment of an indivi-
dual patient and/or his family, according to the
social worker's own method of specialization: i.e.,
casework, group work or community organization.(A
patient writes about his hospital experience: "then,
the social workers are fairly good. Their job is to
keep your family together and eating and they take
you away from your own troubles." [3]) By far, the largest number of social workers have specialized in the

2. Leona Grossman, "The Family of the Patient"
(unpublished paper).

3. Stephen Becker, "On Being a Patient," Atlantic
Monthly, July 1966, p. 98.

casework method and most social workers employed in
health settings are case workers. However, many hospitals with long-term patients (such as the chronically ill), mental and children's hospitals recognize
the value of group work for their patients. Also the
techniques of the group worker have been found to be
applicable with many groups of patients in an acute
general hospital, for example: diabetics, cardiacs,
orthopaedic and various others.

It is interesting to speculate about how very
large hospitals of a thousand beds or more might benefit from the skills of a community organization
worker. These huge, sprawling organizations have a
larger total population including both patients and
staff than many towns and villages, and, like the
towns and villages whose residents are often homo-
geneous economically and socially, the hospital is
a microcosm of many strata. In these mammoth institutions correlation of activities for patients and
staff can become unwieldy; also, in general in large
hospitals to-day, innovations in many areas of the
institution need to be made for effective administration. It is here that a community organization worker
might function, helping to provide a sense of integration for the group within the hospital community
and maintain the focus on the patient.

(b) Collaboration with other members of the
hospital staff to support their services to the patient and to help the patient take full advantage of
medical and nursing care so that he will be able to
use it to regain the maximal level of health and social functioning. Far too often, a patient does not
follow his doctor's advice because of obstacles in
his social environment that must be overcome or re-
moved before he is able to get well. These barriers
to health may be as simple as not having enough money
to buy a brace or as complicated as being overwhelmed
by fear of the future. (For a further discussion of an
aspect of collaboration see below in this chapter.)

(c) Referral to specific community resources
that are appropriate to meet the needs of an individual patient and/or his family. The word to notice
here is appropriate. The social worker uses community
resources in much the same manner as a physician prescribes medication; to explain, a conscientious doctor
does not write a prescription for penicillin for all

patients who have an infection, rather he chooses
the specific antibiotic that is indicated not only
by the disease, but for the patient who has the
disease. Similarly, a social worker does not automatically refer everyone who requires financial
assistance to a public agency. There may be obvious
reasons why a private resource is indicated. Indeed,
it may not be financial assistance which is required
to solve a problem at all. To take what may seem an
extreme case: a patient may be paying blackmail, in
which case legal assistance is the instrument to be
used. He may need simply budgetting help, and there
are several other reasons which could be the cause
of his monetary embarrassment. Community resources
must be used with propriety and discretion in order
to facilitate the alleviation of the social need
and make social treatment possible, thereby enabling
the patient to respond to best advantage to medical
and nursing care.

(d) The social worker normally has enough projects before her to keep her fully occupied, and
does not need to take up research for research's
sake, as has become fashionable in many quarters.
But to be of value, research does not need to be
conducted on a grand scale. There are various groups
of patients or families presenting specific difficulties or needs in every hospital for whom an organized
consideration within a research design might well
find a solution. For example: a research project
might be as uncomplicated as studying methods of
solving lengthy waiting periods for patients in the
admitting office, or it may have such far reaching
repercussions as the research done by the social worker in a Pittsburgh Hospital which resulted in dis-
tinguishing the battered child syndrome that has
stirred doctors, social workers, lawyers and legisla-
tors alike. [4]

2. With the hospital

(a) provision of information both formally and
informally to both professional and non-professional
staff about the implications and meaning of illness
and hospitalization for both a patient and his family.

4. Elizabeth Elmer, "Abused Young Children seen in
Hospitals" (Journal of Social Work, Vol. 5, No. 4,
Oct. 1966), pp. 98-102.

Formal teaching about the social component of illness, its meaning and its treatment, should be a responsibility of the social worker. This teaching can be done within structured lectures and seminars for doctors, interns, nurses, dietitians and others, with the director of the department assigning particular teaching responsibilities to senior workers. In Canada, six medical schools have social workers on staff either full or part time. No information is available as to the number of hospitals with social service departments that are used as teaching centres by the medical schools. But according to a recent survey (1966) of 79 medical schools made by the National Association of Social Workers in the United States, 73 were connected with hospitals where there was a social service department and 31 medical schools have social workers on staff in some unit of medical school. Four other schools stated that they planned to include a social worker on staff in the future. Dr. Clute in The General Practitioner recorded that in Ontario 54.6% and in Nova Scotia 71.4% of the doctors interviewed in his survey were dissatisfied with the course in social work in their undergraduate education. He continued: "social work and physiotherapy both elicited the same comment that there has been little or no instruction in these subjects and that there should be some instruction." [5]

A professionally staffed social service department also has an obligation to provide field work placement for students of social work. (See Chapter IX.)

Within the hospital, the social worker is in an almost perpetual informal "teaching" situation and it can be a fascinating process. Often, she is astonished to recognize that a conversation with an intern over coffee really was informal teaching. However, this process differs from "interpretation" although there may be some overlapping features. Interpretation is also usually done in a less structured way, and may be focussed on a single incident. It may consist of explaining to a doctor why a mother re-

5. Kenneth F. Clute, The General Practitioner: A Study of Medical Education and Practice in Ontario and Nova Scotia (University of Toronto Press 1963) pp. 348-349, 353.

fuses to have a child admitted to hospital, or giving a detailed explanation to an intern why a certain
patient is not eligible for unemployment insurance
and therefore needs a medical report written by him
to make an application for direct welfare assistance.

(b) provision of information and recommendations
to the administrative authority concerning policies
and procedures that affect the social well-being of
the patients, their families and the staff. By being
part of both the hospital and the community, the social worker becomes aware of developments and needs
that affect the social climate of both and can suggest to the administration adjustments in hospital
policies or procedures that will make the hospital a
more effective social instrument. A concrete example:
a hospital in a small town, with a new social worker,
had a large patient population who came from a wide
rural and mining area. Soon, the social worker was
concerned about the loneliness of the patients and
became aware that frequently they discharged themselves against medical advice. A little inquiry
quickly established the reason: visiting hours were
only between 2:00 and 4:00 in the afternoon and were
rigidly enforced. The farmers and miners were unable
to visit during this period; patients thus isolated,
were unable after a certain point to bear the loneliness, so left for home. As a result of the social
worker's findings, the administrator remedied the
situation and morale improved immediately.

(c) Consultation. Social illness, like all other
kinds of illness, is a matter of degree and just as
every sore throat does not need the skills of an oto-
laryngologist so every social problem does not need
the professional help of a social worker. Sometimes,
however, physical symptoms are such that a general
practitioner decides to consult a specialist with
or without the actual examination by the specialist
of the offending throat. The specialist and physician
decide together whether or not the patient should be
seen by the former or simply a different method of
treatment be instituted. Similarly, social workers
offer a consultation service and together with the
person consulting decide whether or not direct social work treatment is needed or only recommendations
for some adjustment. These latter may or may not be
accepted by the person asking for the consultation.

Bartlett in her article "The Widening Scope of Hospital Social Work" says:"consultation should be recognized as distinct from case work and as a valid
professional activity in its own right....Further-
more, it should be clear that consultation may cover
any area of knowledge or practice within the social
worker's competence. It is not limited to patient
care." [6]

   3. <u>Outside the hospital</u>
   (a) Providing information about the social meaning of illness involves responsibilities beyond the
hospital walls and the medical social worker must be
alert to opportunities that present themselves in a
number of areas. Often, a non-medical agency will
ask a medical social worker to talk at a staff meeting about a client it has in her hospital, or an individual worker in the community will need to discuss
in detail a particular family in which a sick member
has caused disruption of the family homeostasis. To
take an example: a senior worker who was asked to
speak at a non-medical agency staff meeting was disturbed to learn how unknowing the workers were about
even common hospital routines; consequently, when
their clients complained, these workers were critical
of the hospital for ignoring the needs of the patients.
Explanation of the need   why routines were necessary cleared up a great deal of misunderstanding and
much animosity disappeared.
   (b) A medical social service department will
normally develop a liaison with the community or
those parts of it that are concerned with the provision of adequate services to meet its health and welfare needs and the use of the services.   Liaison might
involve interpretation to the community about its
hospital and interpretation to the hospital about
the ever-changing community scene. It can also involve identification of inadequate or non-existent
resources and taking action with designated responsible authorities when gaps in services become known.
   We may now turn once again, as promised above
to a discussion of collaboration with other professional staff. Medical social workers are practising
in a setting where the primary goal is physical and

---

6. Harriet M. Bartlett, "The Widening Scope of Hospital Social Work," <u>Social Case Work</u>, Jan. 1963, p.7.

mental health, as distinct from social health, and this very fact obligates them to learn and use skills and techniques that produce effective collaboration. Collaboration in this context may be defined as a process that enables members of different professional disciplines to perform their functions distinctly and separately but with a focus on the achievement of a common goal. The common goal of total patient care is reached when each profession assumes its own responsibility in this activity. Bartlett defines this process as "multi discipline practice" and says "it is a way of thinking, of keeping ideas related, a way of feeling, of readiness to share and a way of doing, of adding one's contribution to that of others so that something larger emerges from the combination. It is a constant interweaving of all these phases of activity." [7]

Social workers in hospitals work in collaboration with doctors, nurses, dietitians and various others, and the method and meaning of collaboration is part of their training. Collaboration cannot by definition be unilateral and is fully effective only when the emotional climate in the organization permits each member of the staff to respect others' professional competence and all have a recognition of a single purpose (in this instance, appropriate and complete treatment of the patient) and of the distinct difference in methods, skills and functions. The degree to which this is possible is determined by many factors, the three most significant being the basic personality structure of the individuals involved, their educational backgrounds, and their past experience.

(a) Doctors. Perhaps collaboration with doctors is the most sensitive of all jointly shared areas both for doctors and social workers. Social workers work closely and directly with both patients and their relatives, and it is the closeness of this relationship that some doctors seem at times to find disturbing. In most instances, this may well be because the doctors concerned do not have adequate knowledge of the professional undertaking of social

---

7. Harriet M. Bartlett, Social Work Practice in the Health Field, (New York: National Association of Social Workers, 95 Madison Ave., New York 16, 1961), p.73.

work. Responsibility for this lack of information must be shared by both medical and social work educators and practitioners. Collaboration can proceed fruitfully when the doctor is able to recognize the social worker as a colleague. A very senior social worker practising in a hospital where the attitudes towards social workers were not noted for friendliness said that one of the bright days of her life occurred when a physician remarked to her that they were in "colleagueship." Dr. John L. Caughey has called the social worker an "associate" of professional status because among other qualifications she has " a special area of knowledge and skill" and "freedom to exercise independent judgment within the assigned area of professional responsibility." 8

Of course, educational experience and attitudes about collaboration are not the only significant factors that determine a physician's openness to collaboration with social workers or others. His concern for people, and his sense of personal and professional security, determine in a great measure too ability to work with others and whether or not he sees in the activity of the social worker a possible erosion of his authority; if he does, he may deny social problems and even reject the worker's skill as part of a professional operation within the hospital. Some doctors have been disturbed because someone other than they has discerned a social problem and referred a patient or his family to a social worker. When this happens a social worker has, of course, an ethical obligation to give help, if it is possible to do so. However, it must be said quickly that social workers have an ethical obligation, equally binding, to consult the physician who is treating the patient and to work in collaboration with him within their own area of competence.

It must be said again that collaboration is not unilateral. Social workers themselves must seek it and endeavour to understand the special responsibilities of doctors and the stress under which these are carried out in today's hospitals.

(b) Nurses. Social workers may find that working with the nursing staff is one of the most satis-

8. John L. Caughey, "Auxiliary Personnel in Medical Practice," (American Journal of Public Health, Vol. 48, No. 8. Aug. 1958).

fying relationships in their hospital experience. However, this again depends both on the nurse herself and the leadership she is given by her supervisors and on the approach made by the social worker.

Frequently, it is the nurse who knows her patients more intimately than anyone and who recognizes the help that the social worker might give because of positive experiences with her in the past. Nurses are busy people, concerned with the immediate demands of the sick and have neither the educational training nor the time to resolve social difficulties that are interfering with the patient's comfort or return to health. Although there are many changes in their educational curricula, their primary focus remains physical care. By mutual sharing of information and recognition of complementary skills, social worker and and nurse can work together in collaborative harmony and the patient is better served. Examples of collaboration between social worker and nurse occur every day and in most instances it is performed by both as a natural happening, without either stopping to think that she is collaborating.

(c) Dietitians; Occupational and Physical Therapists. In numbers they comprise a small percentage of hospital professional staff. There could be many examples of collaboration between the social worker and these other staff members. Two will demonstrate, both of them representing a rather simple incident but meaningful in context.

A seventy-year-old widow with no relatives except a nephew in England was referred to the hospital social worker for help in planning for her care following a lengthy hospitalization because of a coronary. The day before her scheduled discharge the worker happened to be on the ward when her lunch tray arrived and overheard her comment to another patient: "I am a little tired of jello but could eat a pudding." The worker, knowing her to be an undemanding person, offered to ask the dietitian if it were contraindicated by her diet. When the dietitian heard the patient's request, she got the pudding immediately, for which the patient expressed considerable gratitude. That night the patient died. Simple though this incident is, it may be taken as an example of social worker and dietitian focussing on the patient and respecting each other's competence: the dietitian recognizing the worker's methods of individualization and the worker recognizing the dietician's authority in diet.

An example of how physical therapist and social worker can work together is provided by the case of a woman, about forty years old, who was having exercise because of a wrist fracture; this woman brought her four-year-old daughter with her when she came for physiotherapy. The child became so upset every time the therapist touched the patient that she began to suspect something very unhappy in the home that might be resolved by the help of a social worker, and she was right. There was a most complicated social situation and it took many months of social work treatment to alleviate it sufficiently to enable the patient to continue with her physiotherapy until the use of her wrist was regained. The physical therapist and the social worker collaborated closely, adjusting and sharing plans and goals within their own professions as the patient's needs warranted.

IMPLEMENTATION OF THE ROLE AND FUNCTION OF SOCIAL WORK

The service of social work rests on a deep understanding of and a compassion for human beings, a knowledge of how people behave and how they grow, a faith in their capacity to change, and an awareness of their needs and how they are affected by social conditions. If social work in a hospital is to be implemented satisfactorily, these values must be considered by the members of the Board and the Administrator, who must in turn decide whether they will not only support financially, but more significantly, understand and accept the role and function of a social service department and be prepared to be witness to their belief. Perhaps, in the last analysis, it is the Administrator who, half-way between the Board and the Department, has a special responsibility for making social work viable and productive so that patients may be more truly made well. A good comprehension of the discipline of social work and the need for a social worker to retain the identity of her role and functions will be of material assistance in providing circumstances for effective collaboration with all the units (as mentioned above) that make up the hospital setting.

CHAPTER VI

ESTABLISHING AND STAFFING A DEPARTMENT

"This is not the end. It is not even
the beginning of the end. But it is,
perhaps, the end of the beginning!" [1]

In Canada, in 1966, there are 1337 general hospitals,
of which 192 have social service departments. In
the same year in the United States, with 5323 general
hospitals, there are 869 social service departments.
Private hospitals, hospitals for special diseases,
or those operating under government legislation,
such as those administered by the Department of Vet-
erans' Affairs, are not included in these figures.
In either country, [2] however, because social work is
often interpreted flexibly, it is not known how many
of these departments meet professional standards. In
1965, at the request of the Canadian Council on Hospital Accreditation, the Canadian Association of
Social Workers prepared a statement of standards
which are incorporated in the Standards Guide of the
Council and which are to be met before accreditation
is granted. [3] This brief sets out the minimum professional requirements for recognition of the department by the social work profession and when these
are met, evaluation of a department will be possible.
However, in 1966, the Canadian Association of

---

1. Sir Winston Churchil, Speech of the Battle of
Egypt, November 10, 1942.

2. Data from the Canadian Hospital Association,
25 Imperial St., Toronto 7, July, 1965; American
Hospital Association, 840 North Shore Dr., Chicago,
Ill., July, 1965.

3. Canadian Association of Social Workers, "Social
Work in the Hospital" (185 Somerset St.W., Ottawa,
July, 1965).

Social Workers prepared a Statement of Function and Standards of Practice for Social Workers in the Health Field.

The idea that a hospital should have a social service department may be sparked in a variety of ways, but it is usually the administrator who presents to the board and to the medical staff the proposal for the addition of social service. The idea could also originate with a member of the Board, the Women's Auxiliary, or the medical staff. Sometimes, opinion in the community operates as a pressure on the hospital authorities to consider the social effects of illness and hospitalization and their responsibility to provide a service to care for patients' social needs. Wherever the idea originates, any decision to establish a department must receive the approval and wholehearted support of the Board of Directors.

Establishing a department in name and in form may not be so very difficult, but ensuring its productive functioning within the hospital organization can be quite a different matter. The Board members who win approval for their own idea or approve a proposal made by others may have difficulty in giving strong support to the new department because of the remoteness of their contacts and control. This could be particularly so if both the Administrator and the Chiefs of Service have not previously understood and accepted the department as a hospital unit. Once the department is established, a Social Service Committee including Board members as well as doctors, the Administrator and the Director of Social Service, can be very useful in maintaining a liaison (see Chapter VII). However, if the Administrator from the beginning or early believes in the value of social work, understands the role and function of a social service department, and has the support of the Board, its contribution to the care of the patient is ensured. At the same time, interpretation on a sound and realistic basis should be provided for the top echelon of staff whose departments are involved directly in patient care. There may be among them differences of opinion about the contribution of social work, but all should have had access to accurate information about its role and function in the hospital. Because of the specialized nature of this interpretation,

the Board and Administrator would be wise to employ
the services of a medical social work consultant.
Such a consultant can do two things: help with the
provision of interpretation planned for each group
and individual involved, and recommend the actual
first steps to be undertaken before and when a
department is established. Names of available consultants may be obtained from the national professional social work associations both in Canada and
in the United States. Some provincial associations
have a roster of consultants. These experts may be
social workers on the staff of schools or hospitals,
or, in some cases, may be provided by hospital associations or the government body under whose auspices
the hospital functions.

NAME OF DEPARTMENT
    The name of the department might be either
Social Service Department or Social Work Department,
but should not be Social Welfare Department. The
terms social work and social service are inter-
changeable and have the same meaning. The original
term was social service, and the date and reason for
introducing the phrase social work are lost. Octavia
Hill is known to have used the term social worker
and is believed to have been the first to have done
so. One may speculate that in the beginning the emphasis was on the service given, but later, when specific people performed the service on a full time
paid basis, the word worker was introduced to denote
the person. Although they call the staff social
workers, most hospitals designate the department as
Social Service perhaps because the emphasis of the
hospital organization is on service. One notable
exception is Johns Hopkins Hospital, Baltimore,
Maryland, where the department is called Social Work
Department.

BUDGET AND FINANCING
    The costs of maintaining a social service
department are recognized as the responsibility of
the hospital, and the budget for the department is
incorporated into the total budget. It is the responsibility of the director, when she is employed,

to prepare her departmental budget on an annual basis for authorization by the administrator.

The largest proportion of the operating expenditure of the department is for salaries and a meeting of prevailing local salary scales is obviously desirable, and indeed necessary if workers with the necessary qualifications for proper functioning are to be obtained. Scales are established by the profession on the basis of educational preparation, skills, experience and job specifications. Where the operating costs of a hospital are financed by governmental insurance schemes, salary schedules that are allowable costs will be available from the department which has jurisdiction over finance. When these do not coincide with those paid to social workers in local non-governmental agencies, it may be necessary for the hospital to make up the difference from other funds if qualified social workers are to be employed. There are still a few outsiders, although happily in diminishing numbers, who seem to cling to an old conviction about the spiritual rewards of "doing good." In writing about payment to social workers both in America and in England in the 1890's Woodroofe says: "The fact that many accepted payment often incurred the criticism of the rich and the opprobrium of the unthinking. A willingness to work for nothing, it was considered, was the hall-mark of a sincere charity worker." [4] Sometimes an echo of this opinion remains to-day.

The initial budget for the department may have to include sums for the purchase of desks, chairs, typewriters, dictating and transcribing equipment and locked filing cabinets. Office supplies including case folders, white lab coats, and social service crests cost proportionally little. Annually, replacement and addition must be provided for.

PHYSICAL SET-UP

The actual physical location of the department is an important consideration and should be arranged before the department starts operation. For maximum

---

5. Kathleen Woodroofe, From Charity to Social Work (Toronto, 1962), p. 97.

efficiency it is best situated in an area that is
accessible both to patients and to doctors, and in
the vicinity of the out-patient department should
there be one. The point is obvious, but it has
happened that social service departments have been
consigned even to the cellar where the coal used to
be stored. (The author worked once in a basement
laundry converted to social service offices.)

There are differences of opinion as to whether
or not the social workers should have decentralized
offices, or should all work out of a main core but
have reserved interviewing space in clinics and on
the wards. Undoubtedly, experience may provide
different answers, and sometimes, of course, arrangements are determined by actual physical possibilities.
There are practical and psychological considerations
that make a central office the set-up of choice.
When they are able to meet and mingle with members
of their own group, as they go and come from a
central office, the workers in a department can more
easily maintain their focus on social work and be
more aware of their identification with other social
workers. The practical considerations are important
too: secretaries, the master index, records and other
supplies are located most efficiently in the main
office; phone messages and people coming in for ap-
pointments are more sensibly channelled through a
central office.

Offices do not need to be lavish but should be
pleasant if the atmosphere they create is to be in-
viting. Workers need separate offices for interviewing, dictating and study.

The question of physical location may involve
another ramification. There have been many examples
of a chief of a medical service, e.g. orthopedics,
paediatrics or other who feels that better care will
be given to his patients if the administration will
allow him to have a social worker for his service
only. This may happen if the administration and the
chief of service are not fully briefed on the nature
of the contribution a social service department functioning as a whole can make and if the social worker
concerned (perhaps inexperienced) has not had an
opportunity of appreciating the gains for her work
which will come to her by way of departmental
association. Experience is against such an assignment.

ONE DEPARTMENT IN THE HOSPITAL

In the early 1940's, there was a trend to establish separate social service departments within the
hospital based on the assignment to medical departments. In 1960's, amalgamation of these departments
into one administrative unit had come to be considered necessary for good patient care and it often
created a great deal of hard feeling and occasionally
a schism among workers. The National Association of
Social Workers and the American Hospital Association
then made a definitive policy statement that all
social workers should be members of one department.
In 1966, the Canadian Association of Social Workers
incorporated such a policy in its Statement of Function and Standards of Practice. [5]

EMPLOYING STAFF

(a) Director. Interviewing and employing a chief
of any department requires time and patience. Professional criteria are not the only basis on which to
judge the suitability of any applicant; moreover, although objective data such as references are helpful,
they too are only aids. The choice of the director
of the department requires the most careful consideration and wise judgment because it is she who determ-
ines the quality and range of social service in the
hospital organization. It is the director who estab-
lishes the dignity of the department's service and
secures respect for the social treatment of patients,
and she must be able to do this both in respect to
the professional goals and ethics of social work and
to the goal, practices and administrative pattern of
her particular hospital. If she fails to do this,
"the department will become an island not sufficient
unto itself, but limited unto itself, striving for
professional excellence to no achievable end." [6]

5. American Hospital Association, Essentials of a
Social Service Department in Hospitals and Related
Institutions, p. 9.; Canadian Association of Social
Workers, Statement of Function and Standards of
Practice for Social Workers in the Health Field.

6. Beatrice Phillips, "A Director Examines the
Director's Role" Journal of Social Work, (National

The director of a social service department
must have a Master's Degree from an accredited
School of Social Work, [7] be a member of the professional association, and should have not less than
five years experience in a health setting, at least
two of which should have been in a supervisory position. Indeed, some hospitals with large social work
staffs may require that a newly appointed director
have previous experience as director. However, as we
have said, verification of educational and practical
experience is not sufficient evidence for choice.
Personal interview or interviews with the administrator are essential. In these conversations the
administrator will seek and try to assess the degree
to which the would-be director has accepted and is
comfortable with the profession of social work and
her understanding of her own area of competence.
If the social worker does not seem to have integrated
her professional concepts, conflicts are likely to be
inevitable. The social worker, too, will wish to come
to some conclusion about the administrator's acceptance of social work in a hospital setting and would
justifiably be concerned for the future of the department if she felt concern at this stage about the support she might receive. Personalities are important.
The same components of personality that enable a
person to give leadership, work in collaboration,
show tolerance and courtesy obtain for the director
of social service as for the chiefs of other departments. Nevertheless, it is well to remember the
wisdom of the patient who said: "Only angels is per-
fect- and angels ain't born no more."
    All too often, an administrator or members of a
Board complain that they are sincere in their decision to establish a social service department but
are unable to find a suitable person to be director.
All too often, they are right. There is no secret
about the shortage of qualified social workers, and
the profession is not able to offer any propaganda

Association of Social Workers, 2 Park Ave., New York
16), Vol. 9, No. 4, October 1964, p. 93.

7. Canadian Association of Social Workers, "Social
Work in the Hospital."

to the effect that next year or the year after the
supply will meet the demand. This regrettable lack
does not provide easy justification for employing
as director a person with other than professional
qualifications. The problem of finding a qualified
person may perhaps not be in the shortage of social
workers but in the hospital itself. For instance,
the method by which a hospital attempts to find an
applicant for the position of director of social
work may be a significant indication of the readiness of the organization for social work, and the
consequent attraction to it of a qualified person.
Personal contacts and word of mouth advertising in
the proper places are often the most productive
means of recruiting. Other resources are the professional associations and employment services who
know of workers who may be available, or ready for a
change of job. Schools of Social Work and workers in
the field have an informal system of spreading the
news. Advertisements in daily newspapers and professional publications reach a great many, but the
advertisement should be worded with care. An advertisement for a director that reads; "Apply to Personnel Manager," can be an immediate warning that the
hospital is probably not ready for a social work
department. An administrator who understands social
work will see the sense of according the same courtesy to an applicant for the position of director of
social service as he would to any other chief of a
professional department.

Often, an administrator offers a potential
director a position only to have it refused. The
reasons may be obscure to him, but the worker may
have realized that the intramural relationships are
so complicated and the tensions so high that she would
begin a job under difficulties. She may sense an an-
tagonism on the part of other professional staff.
Then again, there may already be an established
department which has not had a desirable complement
of professional workers or where a division has ap-
peared between the workers assigned to the psychiatric
department and the other medical departments. When
any of these circumstances are present, the hospital
may expect to find difficulty in recruiting. There
are well qualified social workers available, and by
and large, they are not afraid of a challenge but

they would be foolishly courageous if they undertook
a job that they knew to have rooted difficulties.

(b) <u>Case Work Staff</u>. It is the responsibility
of the administrator to employ and discharge the
director of the department. The responsibility and
authority for finding, training, and releasing its
staff will, in turn, be hers.

At an early stage the question will certainly
arise, how many social workers? There is one obvious
answer: as many workers as are required to carry the
work load. But there is no rule of thumb or mathemat-
ical formula to determine the number of social workers in relation to number of beds or clinic visits.
The desirable number of social workers can only be
determined as the program of the department develops
and the value of social work skills is recognized and
then utilized more fully by other disciplines. Thus
numbers will be affected by the degree of awareness
of the social aspects of illness that is developed
by the medical and nursing staff, who have the most
frequent and primary relationships with the patients
and their relatives. It is a common experience that
when a social worker is assigned to a service, recognition that patients may be affected by social problems
increases immediately and more patients are referred,
thereby creating the need for more social workers.
A second factor may be the socio-economic level of
community development; the availability of resources
in the community may help or hinder the medical social
worker, and consequently, regulate the amount of work
she must do. Thirdly, if the hospital authorities
expect the social workers to participate in teaching
and research activities to any great extent, more
social work staff is required to carry the basic
function of the department, i.e. social work treatment. And lastly, the degree to which the hospital
is committed to giving comprehensive care to its
patients will determine its expectation of service
from the social workers.

The case work staff should have full professional training and be members of the professional
association. The amount of work experience required
depends on the position to be filled. For example:
a supervisor must be an experienced practitioner,
but less experienced or newly graduated workers
would be suitable for line staff positions.

(c) <u>Social Work Assistants</u>. Social work assistants, case aides, or case assistants, as they are variously called, are being employed in increasing numbers in hospitals where there are large social departments. They have a wide variety of educational backgrounds. In Canada, as has been mentioned in an earlier chapter, a number of technical and community colleges have started courses in social welfare. The students are eligible usually on completion of grade XII (Ontario), and the course of study is completed in two years. Various other educational settings are being used to provide workers in the field including establishing a curriculum in universities with a heavy social welfare content which will lead to a Bachelor of Social Work degree. Summer and night certificate courses are offered by a number of schools. Valuable as these educational opportunities may be, they do not prepare students for full professional activity or responsibility, but as the social work job becomes increasingly complex and different levels of functions and demands begin to be necessary and inevitable, clarification of structured job specifications has increased, and it has been recognized that it is sensible to assign certain functions to persons with less than full professional education. These assistants, some of whom will have an undergraduate degree, can be given on the job training that equips them to undertake responsibilities that add to the contribution of the department but do not require the knowledge and skills of full-scale professional education. They would normally be assigned to assist an experienced senior worker and are carefully supervised in what they are and are not doing in the interests of the patient, of course, and of their own sense of competence. The most appropriate ratio of case aides to trained workers has not been established. This varies with the kind of departmental job to be done and may be determined only by the director. The professional associations are currently studying this situation and, no doubt, will soon make a position statement.

(d) <u>Secretaries</u>. Secretaries and stenographic help are most important in any social service department. The numbers should be determined by the department's needs, and secretaries or clerks assigned to the department with the consent of the director.

The person on receptionist duty, frequently a secretary, is often the first to meet a patient who may
be agitated and upset. A sympathetic and courteous
manner is of the utmost importance, as is a willingness to become involved in the particular goal of
the department and to develop a fitting attitude
to people in trouble.

(e) Volunteers. In the beginning, social work
was done by volunteers, as we have seen in an earlier
chapter. Time passed, however, and to-day, social
work and volunteering are complex activities and are
not synonymous. The volunteer, in any hospital or
health setting, can nevertheless contribute untold
service to the patients (and may actually work directly with them), even though a volunteer, by definition,
cannot do the job of paid staff, and though she may,
in some organizations, work directly with patients.
The reason is not far to seek.   The very nature of
volunteering militates against continuity of care,
regular attendance, and focus on the patient. There
are exceptions of course. This writer has remembered
over a number of years the service of a volunteer,
a trained social worker who, carrying a case load
of cardiac patients, worked every morning for many
years on a volunteer basis (legalities required
that she be paid a dollar a year).

Volunteers, then, are able to perform an infinite variety of jobs that will aid the patients
and the social workers, but these jobs must be clearly defined by the Co-ordinator of Volunteers and the
Director of Social Service. They will normally be
screened, trained and assigned by the Co-ordinator
of Volunteers to the Social Service Department, according to their interests and capabilities. The
director or the staff member who is responsible for
their on-the-job supervision should have an opportunity of approving the placement.

(f) Students. Students are not staff and cannot
be expected to lessen the need for staff. However,
Levin in a new look at "Learning and Teaching in
Field Work" has stated that: "A student who has
qualified for graduate study has as much to give
[the membership] as the vast majority of part-time
staff." [8] For additional discussion of Student

----

8. Morris Levin, "Learning and Teaching in Field Work"

Teaching see Chapter IX.

RE-ESTABLISHING A DEPARTMENT

A social service department or some resemblance thereto may have existed in a hospital organization for many years, even though its role and function have been less than those expected of a professional discipline. Inadequacy or deterioration in the service over time and by the overlay of custom may not be noticed unless a crisis occurs, such as the withdrawal of students by a university, the resignation of a director, or the appearance of a new administrator. Then, questions are asked and the problems are exposed; rehabilitation of such a department can be fraught with complex and frustrating situations, which are, however, not all that different from those found under similar circumstances in other departments. In such situations, the knowledge and cordiality of the administrator toward social work are of primary importance. Final decisions will be his, but he may find an informed committee of the Board a help. A sine qua non, in such situations, is the expert advice of a social work consultant who can study the department and make recommendations for the decision and implementation of the hospital authority. (For criteria for evaluation of a department see Chapter VIII.)

SMALL HOSPITALS

Sometimes the staff of a small hospital (100 beds or less), usually situated in a small community or a rural district, becomes aware of the need of social work treatment for their patients, but do not know how to make it available. There are several possible suggestions, all of which require time and effort to bring to fruition. A hundred-bed hospital might find it advantageous to employ its own social worker. However, if this is not feasible, for a time a temporary expedient would be to investigate the possibility of buying service from the community agencies. Or, several hospitals that are located in

Journal of Jewish Communal Service (National Conference of Jewish Communal Service), Spring 1967, Vol. XLIII, No. 3, p. 270.

the same geographic region might work out an arrangement whereby they employ a social worker on a sharing
basis. This is currently being attempted in Brock-
ville, Ont.

GENERAL RECOMMENDATIONS

Once a department has been established, even
under the best possible conditions, it is wise and
prudent for its director to go slowly. If a great
deal of pressure is exerted on the director to
accept cases immediately, she may find herself doing
so before she or the hospital staff is ready, with
the result that sound policies are not established
and inappropriate jobs are imbedded in the department's functions. In the case of a totally new
department, a director needs time, perhaps two months
of it, to become familiar with the hospital, not only
with the physical structure but with its emotional
climate, its expressed and unexpressed attitudes,
power structures and mores. And the hospital needs
equal time to learn to know and accept her, not only
as a professional person, but as a person. She must
think through and work through policies and procedures making whatever adaptations are necessary for
the particular hospital in conjunction with the Administrator, the various Chiefs of Service, and the
Director of Nursing. When the re-establishment of a
department is involved, proceeding with caution is
an even greater necessity. Time spent attending ward
rounds and conferences, and in discussion with as
many representatives of the hospital staff as possible,
is most productive when the department turns to help
patients.

Experience has also proven that when a department is ready to accept referrals, they should be
taken as they come and not restricted to a particular service. Much is demonstrated in this way: the
staff to whom little interpretation is required will
become evident, the kind of interpretation necessary
in various services can be identified and the numerous problem areas that will require careful handling are defined. Also, from the number and kind of
referrals, the director will get an idea of the
services that are ready for a social worker to be
assigned to them.

The world of most hospitals to-day is a complex
one, and it may be helpful here to touch on some of
the factors which make for complexity and which the
new department must take into account. Number of
patients is one of these. The bed shortage is a
sociological fact. More sick people are admitted to
general hospitals to-day than ever before in history,
because methods of diagnosis and treatment changed
so radically that scientific equipment, much of
which is available only in hospitals, must be used
for accuracy in diagnosis and treatment. Also, frequently patients are covered by insurance payable for
tests only if they are hospitalized. Then again,
physicians, often working under great pressures, find
it much less time-consuming to visit several patients
in hospitals where one stop will do than to drive,
often in bad weather and in the face of parking problems. (Recently, the problem of the non-visiting
doctor has been attracting a great deal of attention
from the news media, particularly magazines and newspapers. The Toronto Daily Star published a series of
eight articles on the situation, beginning March 20,
1967, entitled "Our Doctor Dilemma.") Also, homes
have changed; so have families. No longer are there
relatives or neighbours to care for the sick or convalescent nor is there space in the home to do so.
Sociologists have been examining this facet of the
twentieth century in great detail.

Society, having created these conditions, has
not yet found any method of solving the problems
they present. There is not, and probably will not be,
a sufficient number of beds in nursing homes, convalescent, or chronically ill hospitals, to receive
all the patients who need such accommodation. The
problem is not primarily the social worker's and she
cannot move the patient into non-existing facilities.
However, knowing the problem, she can, in the setting
of her own particular hospital, help its patients to
make most effective use of it and its care and also
help their families to plan for post-discharge care.

Very often, the reasons a patient and/or his
family has difficulty around discharge or post-
hospital care are complex and are not easily discovered; they may include such emotions as that of
an adult who feels guilty about earlier neglect of
a parent, or a wife who can tolerate no longer liv-

ing with her husband. Sometimes, it is lack of or garbled information. For example: An intern talked to a social worker about a wife who refused to take home a patient who was chronically but not acutely ill or severely handicapped. When the social worker talked to the family she learned that both the wife and the son had misunderstood the patient's condition. They loved him very much, but expected him to die any moment and thought that because his death was imminent, he was being discharged from hospital. They were terrified. The solution was simple and immediate; arrangements were made for them to talk to the doctor, who now, understanding the difficulty, clarified the medical situation and the patient was joyfully taken home. Result: another bed. Not infrequently, however, patients are not discharged because of the social worker's recommendation. There are patients who just have no place to go and no one to care for them. Consequently, they must wait in an active treatment bed, either until a bed in an appropriate institution is available or until they are able to care for themselves. Many financial problems will arise, and although these are largely the concern of the business office, they can involve the social service department also. It is not unusual for the social worker to learn that a patient was too embarrassed to admit that he was unemployed or on welfare and had agreed to pay an account that was completely beyond his financial means. Such was the situation of one elderly man who told the clerk in the outpatients department that his son was a pharmacist. Later, when he was asked to pay $2.00 for his medicine, he became very agitated and was referred to the social worker. She learned that although the patient did have a son who was a pharmacist, there had been no communication between them for nearly thirty years. The patient and his wife had separated when the child was an infant, but the lonely old man could not admit this to the clerk. In such circumstances, the worker would recommend to the accounting department that the patient receive free care and her recommendation would usually be accepted.

Social workers may also find themselves involved in following up patients and getting them back to the clinic. Because of the social treatment being given, she may be instrumental in helping a patient to continue medical therapy until he has regained his health and social functioning. By continuing in social work treatment the patient is enabled to complete his medical treatment and thereby reach his individual maximal level of health.

CHAPTER VII

ADMINISTRATION OF THE DEPARTMENT

"In simplest terms, administration is
determined action taken in pursuit of
conscious purpose." [1]

The proper establishment of a Social Service Department complete with staff is only the first step and
does not of itself make a department viable and
productive. It becomes so when the skills and techniques of administration are applied in a way that
enables the social work job to be done well and
ensures the department its place in the over-all
organizational structure of the hospital. The responsibility for the smooth functioning is the director's who will be responsible directly to the Board
through the hospital administration. The person at
administrative level to whom the director reports
may be the administrator himself or his associate
who exercises jurisdiction over all other professional departments. [2]
    Experience makes it necessary to underline the
above chain of command. It avoids the possibility
of the director of social service reporting to someone designated as her authority, but who in reality
has no authority for decision making, and perhaps
no knowledge of what is involved in a decision
affecting social work. It is in these circumstances
that tendencies to view social service as part of
nursing, out-patient, psychiatric or sundry other
departments, and therefore part of their administrative responsibility, can occur, and of course, it
denies the professional integrity of social work
itself.
    The director's function in the administration

1. Fritzmorstein Marx, ed., Elements of Public
Administration (Prentice Hall, New York: 1946),p.3.

2. See Canadian Council on Hospital Accreditation,
Standards for Hospital Social Service Departments.

of her department incorporates all the components of such a responsibility: leadership, organization, program planning, staffing, co-ordination, supervision and evaluation that "translate purpose into action." 3 Also, it requires wisdom, good judgment and courage,   qualities which may not only be learned in the school of experience, but will certainly be enhanced there. Other elements of administrative skills and techniques are also essential.

COMMITTEES
     Committees of several kinds can be valuable adjuncts to the administrative process and, if they are given a definite structure and purpose, the director will find them important aids in her job.
     (1) Intra-departmental Committees.If the staff is large enough, perhaps ten or more members, standing committees of the staff to plan educational projects, review policies and procedures or for other purposes appropriate to the particular hospital and the department would be advisable. In departments with fewer staff members **Ad** Hoc Committees would be more appropriate.
     (2) Extra-departmental Committees. If the administrator agrees and co-operates, an Advisory Committee composed of board members, doctors, and, ex officio, the administrator and director can be utilized in many ways. It is important that the advisory and not supervisory responsibility of such a committee be understood and agreed to by its members.
     A social service committee of the hospital's Medical Advisory Council chaired by a member of the Medical Advisory Council, and with members representing all the medical services, has a tremendous potential for facilitating communication between doctors and social workers. Often this committee, if understanding moves both ways, enables the appropriate and therefore the best use of medical and social work skills in treatment of the patient. With mutual recognition of each other's professional skills, the suggestions and recommendations that this kind of committee can generate must provide better patient

---

3. Fritzmorstein Marx, Elements of Public Administration, p. 121.

care.

WORK ASSIGNMENTS

Work assignments and the supervision and evaluation of the department's work as a whole and the
workers individually, should be provided for within
the department. Number of cases per worker, like
number of staff required, cannot be determined by
the slide rule method. Nor can it be determined by
number of beds or number of clinic visits. There
are many variables that determine a case load. The
number of cases that may be carried effectively by
a worker is related directly to the experience of
the worker, her individual level of performance, her
capacity for organization and her response to pressures. Also it depends on the kinds of problem situations encountered, the availability of community
resources, interpersonal working relationships and
the secretarial or clerical help provided. However,
in evaluating any case load by numbers of cases,
experience has shown that usually, though not always,
cases can be divided into three groups: inactive,
moderately active and very active. For example: at
any given point in time, about one third of a worker's cases require intensive treatment and attention.
Another third will need only some help, and the re-
mainder will have reached a point where only a hold-
ing action is necessary. Needless to say, the emphasis in the cases shifts and there are moments
when a worker has good cause to feel that every case
requires urgent attention.

Work assignments, in terms of areas of responsibility, should be indeed more definite. A worker
should be assigned to a particular medical service
and be responsible for all referrals from both in-
and out-patients on that service, e.g. medicine,
surgery, gynecology, etc... In large hospitals, more
than one worker is needed to give adequate coverage
to a service and so administrative arrangements must
be made with reference to intake of patients. There
are many ways to do this and the ones that are most
effective in any given hospital can be decided by
the director. One of   them would be to assign
intake duty on specific days and responsibility for
all referrals from designated wards to the individ-

ual workers. Also, any patient known to a worker should continue with the same worker, as long as he is the responsibility of the hospital, even though he may be transferred to another medical service. Because all effective social work is family oriented and a large majority of patients come from and return to a family, any member of that family who becomes a patient of the hospital would more effectively be the responsibility of the original worker just as long as this is possible. To illustrate: Mr. X. may be referred from Allergy and seen by the worker, Miss A., in that clinic. Later, he may be admitted for a surgical procedure and be referred again, and while he is still an in-patient, Mrs. X. may be admitted to the Obstetrical ward. It would be best if Miss A., if still on staff, again worked with Mr. X., and with Mrs. X. and any other member of the family as is deemed necessary. Patients experience fragmentation in their medical treatment; surely, they will benefit from continuity in at least one aspect of their contact with hospitals, and it is possible for the social worker to provide that continuity.

POLICY MANUAL AND PERSONNEL PRACTICES

Good administrative practice requires sound and appropriate policies and procedures clearly understandable and recorded in a departmental manual. Indeed every department, not only social service, should have one. Such a book of instructions and regulations takes time to build and assemble and must be revised periodically. Its contents should be explicit about the role and function of the department, the authority by which it operates, personnel policies, management of work loads, general and specific expectations and duties of staff, as well as samples of all forms used in the department. A copy of this document should be on file in the administrator's office and each worker should have her own copy or access to one.

Formulation of personnel policies for any group working in a setting other than a primary milieu is difficult. Professional social work does have clearly defined personnel policies and ethics - so do hospitals. Consequently, flexibility must be ex-

ercised by both the hospital authority and the social
workers to bring these into an agreeable working
alignment. It has been stated by the profession that
the special tensions of a social worker's daily work
require a vacation of four weeks annually, [4] and it
is desirable to adopt this policy as fully as possible. However, some hospitals have a blanket policy
of three weeks maximum holiday. In such circumstances
special arrangements may have to be made. And administrators have been known to be unwilling to make any
adjustment on the basis that in their hospitals some
staff members (such as nurses) get three weeks vacation (although this is not a uniform vacation time
for nurses in all hospitals). Again, all social workers, as do all professional staff, require from time
to time opportunity for study and further education.
Educational leave, as well as time for conferences,
should be given, and this may require special adjustments by the hospital authorities if they are not
customary elsewhere and particularly if financial
help from the budget is required.

It is not feasible to outline details for every
department's operation because of the individual
character of each hospital, and of the variety in
patient populations and in communities. Also, every
director applies administrative techniques according
to her own knowledge and experience, and according
to the need of the department and hospital, adjusting
to the demands of the situation. However, there are
a few basic elements of administration that are necessary to make the department's role active by means
of the department's functions. It is not possible to
give detailed consideration to each one, but a few
will be discussed in the following paragraphs. The
order in which they are discussed is not meant to
indicate priority.

1. Staff Meetings

Staff meetings serve many purposes. They are a
tool of administration; skill in using them demands
thought and carefully used techniques all applied

---

4. Canadian Association of Social Workers, Statement
of Function and Standards of Practice for Social
Workers in the Health Field, 1967.

creatively. They may be used for giving information by the director to her staff, by the staff to their director; they may also be used for sharing information and experiences by staff members, and for policy and procedure planning. They provide an excellent opportunity to have a guest speaker from a community resource, and they may also be used as a device to interpret the job of the department to Board members and other members of the hospital staff. If they are conducted carefully and sensitively, they give the workers an opportunity to express feelings, share frustrations, and air grievances. Observing the interaction between staff members during exchanges of ideas in staff meetings provides the director with an opportunity for evaluating trouble spots in staff relations and disgruntled workers, and may give her a chance to take action before difficulties reach an unsolvable level. The conduct of meetings thus requires thought and creative application of developing administrative skills. Staff meetings should be held at a regularly scheduled time; how often will be determined by the size and activity of the department. Some recommendations are: a full staff meeting including professional and secretarial staff at least once a month, if the staff complement is ten or more. Weekly or bi-weekly meetings are more helpful for smaller staff.

In addition to full staff meetings, casework staff should have their own regular meetings, and in large departments with a number of supervisors they and the director should confer as a group on a weekly basis. This schedule provides an opportunity for sharing, enables the supervisors to obtain a broad knowledge of what is happening in other services, and prevents them and the workers for whom they are responsible from working in isolation.

The educational content of staff meetings may be informal with learning taking place by means of the information and discussion related to items on the agenda. However, this is usually not enough; educational staff meetings should be planned on a regular basis. This programming can be done months in advance with workers assuming responsibility for decisions about the topics to be discussed and the presentation of material relating to them.

2. Supervision

To social workers, supervision has a special
connotation rather different from any it has for
other professional groups. It is a means whereby a
more experienced social worker oversees and guides
a case worker. It is a process that requires a particular technique that may be learned. The beginning
supervisor requires consultation with an experienced
supervisor and, if at all possible, should have a
formal learning experience in supervision given by
a School of Social Work. Depending on the organization of the department, supervisors may have only
supervisory responsibilities or they may combine
supervision and direct practice. A director who is
responsible for supervising three workers does not
have the necessary time to carry a case load. Supervision is significant for two reasons: it is a teaching device and an administrative method. Information
should flow in both directions: from supervisor to
supervisee and from supervisee to supervisor. But
supervision is more than the exchange of information,
it is also a learning experience for both supervisor
and supervisee.
    In the fifties and sixties, there has been a
very strong movement in many agencies and among many
social workers to abolish the supervisory conference.
There have also been experiments with "peer" supervision using group dynamics as the vehicle rather
than the one-to-one relationship used in the traditional method. The professional publications carry
frequent articles on the topic. [5] Various reasons

---

5. For example: here are some articles selected at
random from the Journal of Social Work, published
by the National Association of Social Workers, 1 Park
Ave., New York 16. (a) Ruth Newton Stevens and Fred
A. Hutchinson, "A New Concept of Supervision is
Tested," Vol. 1, No. 3 (July 1956), p. 50; (b) John
Appleby, Virginia Berkman, Robert Blazejack, Vicki
Gorter, "A Group Method of Supervision," Vol. 3, No.
3 (July 1958), p. 18; (c) "Western New York Chapter,
Medical Social Workers Opinions on Supervision, a
Chapter Study," Vol. 3, No. 1 (Jan. 1958), p. 8;
(d) Donald A. Devis, "Teaching and Administrative
Functions in Supervision," Vol. 10, No. 2 (April
1965), p. 83.

in support of abolition of supervision are expressed,
the strongest being that a graduate from a School
of Social Work should be sufficiently competent to
practise without direction. There is sometimes, although it is less frequently acknowledged, an attitude that to be supervised denotes a lower status
in the professional hierarchy. This in reality is
not so; the performances of doctors, lawyers, teachers, administrators and business executives are, in
fact, always under scrutiny in some way or other by
those in whom the final authority in their particular situation rests, even though the supervision
is of an unstructured nature. Supervision is one
way that the supervisor and ultimately the director
has of knowing whether or not the quality of help
meets the required standards. Moreover, supervision
of the proper kind should not be considered only as
surveillance; its intrinsic possibilities of education, information, and policy making should be utilized.

Supervisory sessions should be maintained at
regularly scheduled times, and only a bona fide
emergency should absolve either the worker or the
supervisor from attendance.

3. Ward Rounds

Social workers attend the regular medical ward
rounds with doctors and interns on their services.
Often, during ward rounds, the workers are able to
recognize that a patient has a social problem that
has been overlooked. Rounds also provide an opportunity for the workers to share significant social data
with the doctors and, in their interpretation of it,
to deepen the physician's understanding of any social
factors that may have caused or accentuated the physical breakdown of the patient, or that are preventing
him from making maximal physical recovery. Social
work ward rounds in which the social workers and the
house staff participate can frequently be used to
identify for the intern and resident the social factors affecting the recovery of individual patients
and to discuss and plan with him how the integration
of medical and social treatment may be achieved.
This sharing of discussion within a group can con-
solidate the idea of a team and vitalize the team

approach to the total care of the patient.

4. Records

    The importance of these is seen in the fact that
all hospital records, including those of the social
service department, are permanent documents and may
be subpoened by a court of law and used as evidence.
Beyond this, and more significant in daily use, records are one of the instruments the social worker
uses as an aid in making a social diagnosis, planning methods of treatment and determining treatment
goals.
    The specific format and recording requirements
must be adjusted to the needs of the particular
department and hospital in which they are to be used,
and in terms of the requirements of the department
for teaching and research. Some hospitals use the
unit system and the social work record is included
in the total record. However, even when this is the
custom, some departments keep their own records
separately.
    If separate social service records are kept,
they should contain a family roster, whether or not
the patient is at the time of intake living with his
family, and give other identifying information that
is accurate and current. (It has happened that when
a patient dies, the only address for family or friend
to be found is in the social service record.) If
full social service records are kept separate from
the patient's medical chart, brief notes on the
social worker's activities should be written in both
indoor and outdoor medical charts. Some hospitals
have a system of different coloured sheets in the
medical charts for different departments and, if
this is the established routine, social service
would have its own colour. Some hospitals prefer
chronological recording and, if this is the method
of choice, the social worker's notes should follow
in appropriate order.
    Notes should be clear and concise, and indicate
social diagnosis and treatment plan. Such entries
should be kept current. Locked cabinets for the
storage and protection of information, which is confidential, are essential.
    At present, there is some discussion in the

social work field about the use and cost of records
and some experimentation in other ways of recording
information has been undertaken, but so far no one
seems to have discovered a more useful instrument.
The usual records of a case are costly, in relation
to the worker's time spent in dictation and the
salaries of the secretaries. No doubt, some workers
are carried away by the sound of their own voices
and include a great deal of irrelevant material.
Unfortunately there are others who have almost a
mental block about reporting and their recording
is inadequate and sterile. Until a better vehicle
is discovered, social workers must learn and keep
sharp good recording skills.

Because social records are basically an instrument for use, they must be fashioned to meet
the need. Usually, a department or an agency has two
kinds; they may be called by different names but the
descriptive phrases 'brief service' and 'continuing
case' will indicate the difference.

A brief service is one in which the worker gives
help around a specific need and the whole procedure
is usually completed within a short period of time.
An example of this would be helping a family make
arrangements for temporary care of children during
the mother's hospitalization. It is possible that
in such an activity the worker may become aware of
more serious social pathology, but for any of several reasons decides that it is not appropriate to
undertake a continuing relationship. Nevertheless,
the information must be recorded with appropriate
identifying data, and the record should include a
statement about the other social problems recognized
and the reasons for not giving treatment at that
particular time. An efficient method of keeping this
information is to have it typed on a card, perhaps
5 x 8, and filed for future reference.

A continuing case is rather more complex. It
requires a case folder, a face sheet on which useful
identifying information (such as names of all family
members, current addresses and phone numbers) is
quickly available. The case material should be typed
on white typing paper and the folder should also include all memos and correspondence relating to the
patient or family. The continuing case record is
made when the worker has or expects to have a rela-

tionship with the patient or family over a long
period of time because of many or a severe social
problem that is causing social difficulties. One
such record may occur when a father of a young family becomes chronically ill and the mother has to
assume the roles of both parents; the patient's adjustment to his changed role is difficult and his
ego image is destroyed.

Social records should be available to doctors,
but it is advisable that a social worker be available
to discuss the written material with them. Just as
social workers need a medical interpretation of medical phrases, so do doctors need interpretation of
social work language.

5. Statistics

Statistical information is necessary for the
director and the administrator. A monthly statistical
report would likely include figures for the total
case load itemized to show the number of referrals
and of cases carried over from the previous month
plus a count of interviews both with and for the
patients. ("For the patient" is sometimes called a
collateral interview or visit.) Another figure that
is extremely valuable for administrative use in the
department is the source of referral, i.e. a recording of which individual (doctor, nurse, etc.) recognized a problem that should be referred to social
service for help. Undoubtedly, these sources of referral vary greatly and depend on the kind of hospital,
its staff's awareness of social problems, their significance to the patient, the possibility of help being
provided by the social workers, and the level of community development in providing for social needs.
Usually referrals from doctors, nurses, relatives,
community social agencies and self, predominate.
Other important information for the director to have
is the percentage of patients referred from the different medical specialities. This is indicative of the
measure of understanding of the personnel of the
various services, and points out where further interpretation is required as well as the services on
which patients may not be receiving total care. An
annual statistical report, which summarizes the
monthly reports, should be required by the admin-

istration and, hopefully, used in the annual report of the hospital. Statistics are valid of course only if the constants on which they are based remain constant. For example: "the case" integer cannot be reckoned at one time as a patient and at another as a family unit. Number of referrals cannot be counted by totalling only new cases in one year, i.e. patient not previously known to the department, and by total-ing <u>all</u> referrals including new cases and those already known but re-referred.

Individual workers are responsible for their own monthly statistical report. These individual reports should be totalled and a copy sent to the administrator and one kept on file in the department. Each department must design its own statistical form according to its needs with full realization that there is no virtue in collecting figures for them-selves. They must be usable and used.

6. Narrative Reports

Statistical reports submitted at monthly and annual intervals provide the director and hospital administration with essential figures that are in-dices of trends, lacunae, patient care and, perhaps, staff competence in using the total resources of the hospital. But these are only a skeleton that should be fleshed by a narrative report that describes not only what has been done for patients, but why it was done, what hospital and community resources were employed, and how collaboration was achieved. Often, the inclusion of a summary of work with a patient with identifying data carefully disguised, makes the role and function of the department and the hospital more graphic than any amount of figures. These nar-rative reports should include happenings that are both sad and joyful, unsuccessful attempts at help as well as those with a satisfactory ending.

The astute director of Social Service is well advised to prepare at least bi-monthly brief narra-tive reports for the administrator and the members of the Social Service Committee, if one exists. An annual report including a summary of both the year's statistics and the happenings in the department (teaching, committee participation, and changes in program) is of great value. It should have as wide

distribution as is discreet to such people as Board
and Auxiliary members, medical staff and appropriate
community agencies.

7. Emergency Service

     Most social agencies have found it necessary
to provide a 24-hour, 365-day service on an emergency basis. Many cities have organized a central
clearing service for social emergencies after hours
and on holidays. Hospital social service departments
should offer the same round the clock service. In
the Massachusetts General Hospital "the emergency
service was instituted which dealt primarily with
life or death situations. In recent years, this is
no longer true. Approximately 50% of the admissions
are now social or psychiatric problems rather than
medical." [6] Social emergencies due to sudden illness
simply cannot be planned; a young mother's life may
depend on immediate admission to hospital at mid-
night Saturday, but she may consent only if she knows
the some responsible person can be located to care
for her three pre-school children. Or, an elderly
man caring for a paralysed wife may require hospitalization on a holiday because of a coronary, but may
refuse unless he has some one to look after "the
missus."
     Consequently, every social service department
in a hospital should have a schedule of workers on
emergency duty. This list should be posted on the
main switchboard. Anyone requiring a social worker
would then call operator who can take the name and
phone number of the person calling, locate the worker on duty and relay the information. It is then the
worker's responsibility to do whatever is necessary
to deal with the emergency.

8. Forms, Equipment, and Clothing

     Without knowing the specific requirements of a
department, it is not possible or wise to make any
suggestions or offer a judgment about the number of

6. Elinor Clark, "Round the Clock Emergency Psychiatric Services" in Crisis Intervention, Howard J. Parad,
(New York: Family Service Association of America,
1966), p. 262.

forms or the kind that may be required. However, it
is possible to say that the fewer the better. If a
form is required for a particular purpose, it must
ask for information in sufficient detail to make it
useful -- it should not ask for bits of unrelated
information or information that would logically be
recorded in another place. For example: a form that
asks about wages is valid only on the day it is completed. When it is significant, the financial situation of a patient should be recorded in the body of
the record about him and changes be noted as the income changes.

So, in the matter of developing forms, each
department must establish procedures that are most
useful to its needs and its staff. However, the
master index form must be given special attention.
It is especially mentioned here because some departments (some of them large) have been known not to
have one, and confusion and inefficiency can result.
No department can really operate efficiently without
one. This card system must be kept up-to-date and
should have readily available necessary identifying
data including current addresses and phone numbers,
as well as case number and whether or not the case
is opened or closed. A very simple but adequate one
is illustrated. The family roster is typed on the back.

Social service requires nothing expensive or

```
+--------------------------------------------------------------+
|                     MASTER INDEX CARD                        |
| NAME........................... CASE NO...........           |
| MAIDEN NAME .................... DATE OF BIRTH....            |
| ADDRESS ........................ TELEPHONE NO ....           |
| .............................................................|
| .............................................................|
| OPENED ......... RE-OPENED...... RE-OPENED........           |
| CLOSED.......... CLOSED ........ CLOSED ..........           |
| RE-OPENED....... RE-OPENED...... RE-OPENED .......           |
| CLOSED.......... CLOSED ........ CLOSED ..........           |
+--------------------------------------------------------------+
```

elaborate in office equipment. Individual offices
and desks, telephones, dictating and transcribing
machines, typewriters, paper and pencils, and the
occasional box of facial tissues are the social
workers' professional instruments other than themselves.

It is desirable that the social service workers
have white coats. These may be in the latest labora-
tory style, but with "Social Service" woven in some
easily visible spot, perhaps on the upper arm. The
white coat labelled "Social Service" identifies them
as belonging to the hospital and signifies their
role and function. Although some hospitals require
social workers to wear white uniforms, this is really
unnecessary, and indeed, it is time consuming for
them to have to change when they have to make home
visits. Also there is a psychological subtlety in
the white coat over street clothes. The social worker
is the member of the hospital staff working with the
patients who represents both their care in the hospital and their resumption of living in the community. Some departments like their workers to wear
name plates and this is a matter of the individual
department's choice.

CLOSING CASES
Often questions are raised, and rightly so,
about the length of time patients are given help
by a social service department. Usually a patient
becomes known to a social service department because
he has a problem of social adjustment that has been
caused or made more severe by his illness, and in
these situations, the responsibility of the social
worker is clear. The case will be closed when social
functioning has been restored or reached a level
with which the patient is satisfied. However, sometimes patients who have social problems not connected
with their illness are referred. Here the diagnostic
skills of the social worker are most important in
planning social treatment in these cases and in using
community resources appropriately. Consequently, if
the illness is the disrupting factor that caused or
exacerbated the social condition, the patient and
family must be the responsibility of the social
worker until both physical and social dysfunction

have either   been resolved or have achieved a
homeostasis. If the problem is not related to the
illness, referral should be made to the community
agency that is able to provide the necessary help.
However, simple referral is not enough; the medical
social worker is responsible for the patient until
the referral has been accepted and acted upon by the
other agency. These criteria must be used with discretion, of course, with the welfare of the patient
and his family being the central concern at all times.

COLLABORATIVE AND CO-OPERATIVE SOCIAL WORK
     Collaboration and co-operation with community
agencies are two processes in social work practice
that merit consideration in medical social work because both the patient and the hospital are in and
of the community and neither can exist without it.
There should be little difficulty in comprehending
their value and their use. In collaborative work,
several workers representing several agencies may
be working with the same family or with the same
person. In this instance, the area of responsibility
of each must be defined clearly, usually in a conference attended by all involved. For example: Mr.
B. may be a cardiac patient, known to the medical
social worker because he cannot accept his physical
limitations. His son, Billy, may be under the care
of Big Brothers, and the whole family known to the
family agency for marital counselling and budgeting
help. The role of each agency in this example is
abundantly clear and each worker should function
in relation to her role, at the same time sharing
with the others developments that affect the whole.
     Sometimes, a little co-operation between social
workers from different agencies is all that is needed but, again, the decision for this method of working with a patient or a family may require a conference. Usually, in co-operative work, one agency
maintains the responsibility for treatment with
another agency providing a necessary service that
could not be obtained otherwise. An illustration
of this might be when a patient on a diabetic diet
who is being helped by the worker in the hospital
to accept the necessary adaptations in his life
pattern requires money to buy the prescribed foods.
A department of public welfare or some specialized

organization may supply the extra dollars, but the
case work service remains with the medical social
worker.

CASE CONFERENCES
     Case conferences are those in which all those
who are working directly with a patient or his
family meet together, share information, define
areas of responsibility and plan goals. This thinking and planning together may be one of the most
productive uses of time in terms of helping a patient that staff can undertake.
     These conferences may be attended by members
of the hospital staff including doctor, nurse,
physical therapist, social worker and others who
have a direct relationship to the treatment of the
patient being discussed. This is a regularly scheduled procedure in some hospitals and on some medical
services. Or, the conference may include hospital
personnel, hopefully the interested doctor, and
also representatives from all the community agencies
who are involved.
     In areas where medical social work is in the
early stages of development, or where it is not well
accepted in the community, these conferences have
several values. The patient is better served and
the workers from the community agencies learn both
about the resources within the hospital and about
the role of the social worker in the treatment of
the patient. If a doctor participates, he will be
made aware of the resources that he can call upon
when his patient needs them.

CONFIDENTIALITY
     Social workers, from the earliest days of their
training, are imbued with their responsibility in
keeping secret information entrusted to them in the
client-worker relationship. There are a great many
facets to this concept which have engaged the attention of social workers over the years. Alves defines
it as "an ethical principle that is related to the
conduct of the caseworker throughout the professional
relationship with a client. Observation or violation
of the principle is possible (1) in the process of

obtaining secret or confidential information about
clients, (2) in the process of recording it, (3) in
the divulgence of it to others." [7] Richmond, in What
is Social Casework? [8] published in 1922, is most
specific about the social worker's responsibility to
keep information confidential. The Code of Ethics of
the Canadian Association of Social Workers states
the professional position as also do several of their
documents. Perhaps one of the most comprehensive and
worthwhile references on the subject is the doctoral
dissertation Confidentiality in Social Work by Joseph
T. Alves, [9] quoted just above.

Consequently, medical social workers are gov-
erned both by their own professional Code of Ethics
and by that of the hospital. Both must be observed.
When a question of legality arises, since hospital
social records are subject to sub-poena, it must be
taken to the Administrator for his decision. Sometimes, amusing and disconcerting situations can happen. A social worker may guard most carefully some
items of information confided as a deep, dark, and
shameful secret by a patient, only to find that
other patients, and often the neighbours, know more
about it than she does.

Nevertheless, social workers must know their
obligation to respect confidentiality and share only
information that is pertinent to the treatment situation. Sometimes this sharing may have to be done without the patient's consent or even against his wishes.
If a social worker puts the full responsibility on
the patient for a decision as to what should be shared,
she is really abrogating the responsibility

7. Joseph T, Alves, Confidentiality in Social Work
A dissertation (Washington, D.C.: Catholic University of America Press, 1959), p. 118.

8. Mary Richmond, What is Social Case Work? (New
York: Russell Sage Foundation, 1922), p. 29.

9. Joseph T. Alves, Confidentiality in Social Work;
see note 7.

that accompanies her professional knowledge and experience. It would be similar to a doctor saying to
a patient in severe shock because of a hemorrhage
"Wouldn't you like a transfusion?"

JOBS WHICH MAY OR MAY NOT REQUIRE SOCIAL WORKERS
     There are activities in any hospital that are
essential both for the operation of the hospital
organization itself and for the welfare of the patient, but they do not require social work skills
for their performance. Nevertheless, in some hospitals, perhaps because of custom, pressure or ignor-
ance of the social work function, these have been al-
located to the social worker. Because she may be
anxious to establish herself in the hospital family,
she may take on jobs that do not fit her skill and
job responsibility. There could be a danger of the
social work function being crowded out and a consequent dissatisfaction with Social Service and even
a re-evaluation of it. Among these jobs are routine
interviewing to establish financial eligibility,
locating another kind of institution for post-
discharge care, and the completion of sundry forms.
     Each and every one of these procedures is ne-
cessary but it is not efficient to use for them the
expensive time of professional social work staff
who may not even have the appropriate skills and
techniques. These tasks would be more competently
performed by other personnel trained for this purpose. However, these persons may well discover or
suspect a social problem in certain cases and they
should be sufficiently aware of the possibility
that social problems can exist and how to refer the
troubled person to a social worker. To illustrate a
situation where an apparently straightforward financial matter became more involved: a mother brought
an insurance cheque to the hospital cashier to pay
for her son's hospitalization which was the result
of a car accident. The cheque required signature of
both the hospital and the parents, but the mother
asked the cashier to give her the money and allow
her to pay the bill in five dollar monthly instal-
ments. When the cashier explained why this arrangement was not possible, the mother burst into tears
and said that she really needed the money to feed

her family -- whereupon the cashier took her to see a social worker. The home situation was sad indeed; the husband and father was unable to keep a job because he was mentally ill and was refusing any kind of psychiatric help. The mother was struggling to keep the family together by doing such work as she could find. She was completely unskilled and her income was less than minimal.

It is recognized that although every patient whose condition requires that he be transferred to another kind of institution for further care, whether convalescent or long term, experiences social and emotional dislocation to some degree, most are able to accept the change without significant distress. In these simple straightforward situations, the staff doctor or his intern can have the necessary application for transfer forms readily available on the floor, complete them, and send them to a suitable hospital employee (such as a clerk), who will get in touch with the possible resources and make the necessary arrangements for the transfer. A recommendation for additional care is as much part of the doctor's prescription for treatment as is his prescription for drugs. However, all planning for post-discharge care is not so uncomplicated. The patient may reject any thought of going any place but home; the relatives may decide they won't take him home, or the cold reality may exist that home is a lonely third floor room and no place for an elderly cardiac patient. In these and similar circumstances, completion of the transfer papers is not enough. They remain within the province of the physician, but the social worker's skills are required to facilitate their use.

In every organization, there are odds and ends of jobs that seem to belong to nobody, but must be done to assure the smooth functioning of the whole. The administrative responsibility of the Director of the Department should include evaluation and decision within the framework of social work as to those that are undertaken by the Social Service Department.

CRITERIA FOR EVALUATION OF A SOCIAL SERVICE DEPARTMENT

When it becomes necessary, and it may for any of a number of reasons, to evaluate the organization and performance of a social service department, the hospital authority would be well advised to employ the services of a social work consultant. In fact, the use of a consultant in such circumstances cannot be recommended too strongly. Criteria for such an evaluation are not easily defined in detail, except as they pertain to individual situations. The following scheme for such an evaluation is suggested as an outline for investigation but does not claim to cover all points that should be considered:

1. What are the professional qualifications of the director and staff?

2. Are departmental policies and procedures outlined in a manual?

3. Are there regularly scheduled times for supervision, staff meetings, and evaluation of performance?

4. Is the proportion of brief services to continuing cases more than one-third of the total case load?

5. What is the quality of social work treatment? To what extent are social needs being met?

6. Are records properly made and kept up-to-date?

7. Are monthly statistical reports kept and submitted to the administration?

8. How are the workers accepted by others in the hospital?

9. What kind of relationship do they have with other staff?

10. Does the staff participate in hospital activities and programs, such as teaching other disciplines?

11. Does the professional staff participate in community action related to health and welfare?

CHAPTER VIII

SOCIAL PROBLEMS DON'T GO AWAY

"We are the hollow men
We are the stuffed men
Leaning together." [1]

Social problems don't go away by themselves, at
least, most of them don't. But when social work
treatment can be given to the individual (patient)
who has them, many can be resolved or their severity
lessened. The frequent complementarity of illness
and social problems has been well studied and well
documented; every library has a great deal of reference material on the subject. And there is no
longer any real dispute as to whether or not family
and relatives suffer disruption in the social aspects
of life when one of their members becomes sick and
is hospitalized. The crisis produced by illness and
the change in family stability is identifiable. It
can awaken old problems, change life systems,
threaten roles and demand a redefinition of values
and faiths. Bloom remarks: "The drama of family life
is perhaps nowhere given fuller expression than in
illness." [2] However, not all persons under severe
and sudden stress break down, nor is the degree of
a break or disintegration related necessarily to the
kind of stress. Consequently, not every patient who
has a social problem needs social work treatment, [3]
but if he does, he will suffer if he is not given it.
    This chapter presents examples which have been
included to demonstrate the range of social problems
that may affect an individual's health, his reaction
to illness, and his capacity to use medical and nurs-

1. T.S. Eliot, "The Hollow Men."

2. Samuel W. Bloom, The Doctor and his Patient
(New York: Free Press, 1965), p. 135.

3. Margaret Brock, "The Doctor and the Social Worker,"
Canadian Medical Association Journal (Sept. 23, 1961),
Vol. 85, p. 749.

ing care effectively, and which consequently require social work treatment for resolution. In no
way do they represent a complete picture of the
social problems that confront patients, their families, or social workers whose major function is
the treatment of such problems (see Chapter V).
Each shows a different facet of the meaning of illness in relation to the difference in the individual's adjustment to illness; no attempt has been
made to focus on the skills and techniques of the
worker.

It must be emphasized strongly that all identifying data in these histories have been changed.
However, these patients did exist and their problems
were real. It will be obvious that the relation of
the histories here gives but the skeleton of the
situation and that only salient facts are presented.

A LOSS OF SELF-ESTEEM

Mrs. Stone, a married woman of 58, was admitted
to hospital for control of hypertension. The nurse
referred her to the social worker because she "cried
too much." The worker found her to be an intelligent,
well-educated woman who responded quickly and warmly,
but who felt useless and a burden to herself and her
family because of a severe loss of vision which had
begun about two years earlier. Now, the patient was
able only to distinguish moving objects and light
from dark.

About the same time as the patient began to lose
her sight, her husband had retired and they moved
from their home in the city, where their two married
children lived, to a small town forty miles away.
Since the change in their living conditions, the
patient had suffered from increasingly severe hypertension. Prior to the move and the onset of her blind-
ness, she had been very active in church and welfare
organizations and with social activities, and was
very close to her two sons, their wives, and their
children. Now she was isolated. She was unfamiliar
with the house, the community, and the people living
there. Consequently she just sat. She was unable to
read, to visit, or do many of her household chores.
Mrs. Stone confided in the worker that she was so
depressed that she wanted to cry all the time.

However, she did her best to withhold her tears
until her husband was asleep and then spent many
hours weeping.

The worker discussed with Mrs. Stone the resources of the Canadian Institute for the Blind
and found her eager for this help. She then talked
with the doctor and Mr. Stone to obtain their collaboration in working out more satisfactory daily
living experiences for Mrs. Stone. The next step was
to arrange a visit by a worker from the Canadian
National Institute for the Blind to the patient while
she was in hospital. This worker, who would keep in
touch with her when she was discharged from hospital,
made plans to get Mrs. Stone records from their large
library of books and music, obtain a Braille teacher,
and provide the many household aids that enable blind
and partially sighted individuals to do most of their
house work. Almost immediately the patient's condition began to improve; she became better able to care
for herself and acquired some housekeeping techniques
to replace those she had lost with her sight. With
a new vitality of interest, she gradually regained
a feeling of worth.

A COMPLEX OF NEEDS

Mr. Rawson, age 51, was referred by the doctor
because he said he could not afford to buy a drop
foot splint. He had a paralysis of unknown etiology.
Provision of the appliance was not difficult, but
the worker then learned that Mr. Rawson's paralysis
was expected to progress, that his only work skills
were those of a waiter, that he had been unemployed
for six months and for three months had been living
on handouts from friends and relatives, and that his
wife, age 49, was confined to bed because of a back
injury and was without any medical care. The immediate needs received first attention, i.e. the splint,
and assistance from public welfare and medical care
for Mrs. Rawson were quickly obtained. The near future would have to include job re-training for the
patient.

INVOLVEMENT OF OTHERS

Bob Simpson, a 14-year-old boy in grade 7, was

referred by the physician in clinic because his
mother had complained he was not doing well at school.
He was physically in good condition but had infantile
speech. Social work treatment for Bob would involve
parents, siblings, school teacher, and speech therapist. Bob was a sensitive boy, rather larger than
his peers, of above average intelligence, interested
in music, but very much overlooked in all the family
affairs. Because he was shy and embarrassed by his
speech, he faded into the class and his teacher
ignored him. His father, a tense salesman, prone to
quick tempers,controlled the home. Mrs. Simpson was
well meaning but needed help to cope with this problem. The younger siblings teased Bob, as did his
classmates. Mr. Simpson was seen only twice, once in
the home and once in the worker's office -- he was
"too busy." Obviously, the family's method of handling the situation was compounding Bob's problem.
Bob was encouraged by the worker in his music and
to express what he felt was the problem in his relationship with his family, his teachers and his brothers. He began to talk over with his worker his method of handling his difficulties and what he felt
about school. Mrs. Simpson was given the same kind
of help and when the worker visited the school, he
was given a warm reception and the teacher was willing to listen, understand, and co-operate. When Bob
was ready, arrangements were made for speech therapy.
When the case was closed, he had made such progress
that he had lost his infantile speech, had obtained
excellent grades in school, was taking guitar less-
ons and had made a friend of a boy who had similar
interests. Although Mr. Simpson could not express
his deepened understanding, he reported that family
life was less hectic.

PROGNOSIS -- NEGATIVE
     Mr. Nagy, age 62, was admitted to hospital and
diagnosed as an advanced gastric carcinoma. He was
referred to social service by his employer who phoned
the social worker because he was worried about Mrs.
Nagy. This childless couple had moved to a new city
only two months before Mr. Nagy's illness and had
been employed as houseman and housemaid. They had
emigrated from Europe six years earlier and had

settled in X city, where Mr. Nagy had attempted to
run a restaurant but had been unable to make a
success of it because of difference in language and
in customs; he had decided to try a new city and a
new job. When the worker talked with Mr. Nagy on the
ward, she found him to be intelligent and co-operative. He spoke excellent English, but was greatly upset about his wife whose English was limited and who
had had both a coronary and a depression, and who
was now living alone in a room without any financial
resources. Mr. Nagy's condition became critical and
he died; but during the two months of his illness,
the worker had almost daily contact with Mrs. Nagy
who became completely immobilized, almost to the
point of being mute. Frequently, all she required
was that the worker hold her hand. One week-end,
when the husband was unconscious, Mrs. Nagy and the
worker walked the streets for hours. The only service
that was concrete and possible was to obtain financial
assistance for her. When she would allow the worker
to do so, the latter got in touch with a friend in
X city who came to be with Mrs. Nagy for the funeral.
She persuaded her to return to X city where she had
a few, if tenuous, roots.

EFFECTS OF MISINFORMATION
     Mrs. Holst, an immigrant to Canada, was referred
from diabetic clinic because the doctor was unable
to make any sense of her weeping and lack of control.
She was 32 years old and had two children, a girl 4,
and a boy 2. Mr. Holst, age 45, was employed and the
income was adequate. Mrs. Holst's diabetes, diagnosed
a month earlier, was mild and the doctor expected
that it could be controlled easily by modification
of diet and medication; he had given her this interpretation. However, she came to clinic every week in
a hysterical condition and was deteriorating rapidly.
When the worker asked Mrs. Holst why she didn't be-
lieve the doctor, she burst into tears again and said
that the doctor was just being nice -- she herself
knew she was dying. Then the worker learned that this
emotional reaction was because, sometime in the past,
when she had been hospitalized in her homeland, two
women who had been in her ward had died. She had been
told that they had "diabetes;" now she too had

diabetes and inevitably she was dying. She believed
this so firmly that she had said farewell to her
husband and children and had written to her sister
in Europe to come immediately to take care of her
children. Doctor and social worker combined their
efforts and Mrs. Holst was finally persuaded to be-
lieve the truth about her condition. She cancelled
her plea to her sister and six years later was in
excellent health.

WHEN THE PATIENT IS NOT THE PATIENT
       Mrs. Adams was a frequent visitor to medical
clinic with multitudinous aches and pains. Extensive
investigation revealed no physical disease. One day
she asked the clinician for work, and was sent to
the social service department. Mrs. Adams' problem
was two psychotic teen-aged daughters. One frequently locked herself in her room; the other wandered
the house at all hours of the day and night with the
result that Mr. Adams was spending his time with
another woman living down the street. It took about
six weeks to have both girls committed to a mental
hospital. After treatment, one was discharged and
made a fairly good adjustment. The other was also
discharged but had frequent periodic exacerbations
and required re-admission to the mental hospital.
However, Mrs. Adams' pains disappeared, Mr. Adams
came home, and Mrs. Adams was able to accept help
in re-building a life for herself with no more than
the normal amount of aches and pains.

INTERNATIONAL IMPLICATIONS
       After three weeks' hospitalization Mr. Downey,
age 60, died. Because his admission sheet showed no
relatives or friends, and the doctors wanted authority for an autopsy, his death was brought to the
attention of the administrator who in turn went to
the social service department. Working only from an
address at first, the worker learned that Mr. Downey
had lived on public assistance for ten years, that
he left his room infrequently, and had no friends.
His landlady did know that he had a sister in his
native country with whom he corresponded at about
five-year intervals. With the help of the Inter-

national Red Cross, the sister was reached, gave
permission for the autopsy, sent funds to have the
body cremated, and requested that the ashes be sent
to her for burial. Also, the worker learned that Mr.
Downey had never married, that he had been a prize-
fighter in his youth, had a prison record, and that
his sister had not seen him for forty years. While
the autopsy was being done, the worker got in touch
with the Trade Commission of Mr. Downey's homeland
and the undertaker. The latter was most helpful and,
when he learned the circumstances, reduced his fee
to the minimum. However, the money sent by the sister
was not sufficient to cover the costs and the deficit
was made up by the Trade Commission.

It is unfortunate that someone did not realize
Mr. Downey's deep loneliness while he was alive, but
the efforts of the social worker undoubtedly helped
ease the pain, perhaps life long, of Mr. Downey's
relatives, and certainly furthered a good international feeling because somebody, i.e. the hospital,
cared.

HOSPITALIZATION AND CULTURAL DETERMINANTS

Mario Colanti was very young, both in age (23)
and in maturity. Nevertheless, he had sought his
fortune in a strange land with a very young wife. He
had had rheumatic fever as a child and about a year
after settling in his new country, when his son was
two months old, he became ill and had to spend nine
weeks in a large modern hospital. He saw the worker
on the ward and asked to talk to her (self-referral)
because he wanted to go home: his wife had no money.
This was a problem, but one that could be solved
without too great difficulty. However, as the worker
continued the relationship with Mr. Colanti, other
problems no less real but more difficult of resolution became evident. Mr. Colanti was gradually becoming adjusted to a completely different socio-economic culture, partly because of his contacts in the
factory where he worked, and because a few of his
boyhood friends from his native village had emigrated with him, but Mrs. Colanti had not begun to become accustomed to a totally different society. She
was very lonely and had not been able to learn English, nor could she understand North American ways

of shopping, telephoning, or even church affiliation. Indeed, because of the infant, she had had very little opportunity to make friends, and with Mr. Colanti's hospitalization in a frightening and to her monstrous antiseptic institution, she was overwhelmed completely. The situation was further complicated because she had no one with whom she could leave the baby while she visited her husband.

The worker's activities in this case were many and were not directed simply to immediate practical solutions, such as using social service funds to pay for a baby sitter. Using her knowledge of human dynamics, she helped Mrs. Colanti to become less frightened of the hospital and its doctors and nurses, and less fearful about shopping; she supported her in making arrangements to learn English at a Settlement House and attend a Well Baby Clinic. All went well until about six weeks after Mr. Colanti's hospitalization, when he became increasingly depressed. One day the worker found him in tears. He said he knew he was dying. This came as a surprise because, in fact, he had made better than expected progress and the worker knew that the doctor had told him so. But neither the doctor nor the worker had understood the reason that the patient had asked for repeated assurance about getting well. The day of the tears, the reason was expressed. When somebody went to hospital in Mr. Colanti's country, friends and relatives visited only as long as there was a possibility of the patient's recovery. When Mr. Colanti was first admitted, he had frequent visits from his few friends but for the past ten days nobody had been to see him; therefore he was dying and he was steadfast in his belief that the doctor's words of assurance and encouragement were only kindness although he hesitated to tell the doctor that he thought so. He found it very difficult to comprehend that the pressure of highly urbanized living interfered with friends visiting the sick over a prolonged period of time. It took many hours of interpretation and support from both doctor and social worker to lift the depression.

ILLNESS AND MARITAL EQUILIBRIUM
Following a colostomy, Mr. Smith, age 57, was considered by doctors and nurses alike as "unco-

operative" because he refused to learn to do his
irrigations and to adjust to hospital routines,
and was "demanding." But this behaviour, as often
happens, was only symptomatic of underlying social
pathology. He was referred to social service because
each time the doctor discussed discharge with him,
he developed numerous physical complaints which, however, could not be substantiated by examination. Mr.
Smith's social service record is lengthy because over
an eight-month period the worker had weekly interviews with both Mr. and Mrs. Smith, frequent dis-
cussions with the staff doctors and the resident,
two out-patient department clinics and three social
agencies. Mr. Smith finally learned to accept his
illness and looked forward to returning to his job
as a taxi driver. Mrs. Smith was helped to accept
the fact that Mr. Smith was going to survive and
recover, and that he would be around the house more
than before his surgery. Under all Mr. Smith's "unco-
operative" behaviour was a precarious marital adjustment, the equilibrium of which had been upset by his
illness. He was difficult in hospital because he did
not want to go home to a wife who didn't want him.
She had not wanted him when he was well and able to
be out of the house 15 to 18 hours a day; undoubtedly
she didn't want him now. This couple had found their
own solution to an unsatisfactory marriage that worked
just as long as illness did not disturb the balance.
      Mrs. Smith was an attractive, intelligent woman,
whom life had disappointed. Nevertheless, she cared
for her home and two teen-age sons (who gave every
evidence of being relatively stable boys and good
students) in an excellent manner and had developed
her own friends and hobbies. Mr. Smith, who was some-
what less intelligent, had fashioned his own life: he
drove his taxi and spent his spare time with his
friends out of the home. Until social work help was
given them, neither could face the changes that illness had forced upon them.

WHERE HELP IS NOT POSSIBLE
      The ideology of professional social work remains
based, as it always has been, on a stubborn optimism
that individuals can be helped to change, to live
lives that contain more satisfaction for them, lives

that are more productive in terms of the community.
But there are times, all too many times, when efforts
to help seem to fail. The reasons for failure or an
unsatisfactory outcome are many and complex; some
are inherent in the combination of the particular
personality of the patient and the particular problem.
Others, of course, may be related to the level of
development of the skills of the worker, to the knowledge that is available at any point in time, or to
the actual length of time there is for treatment.

A few examples will illustrate these kinds of
"mission difficult" or "mission impossible."

(a) Unreasonable Demands

Sylvia Myer, age 55, divorced ten years ago
after four weeks of marriage, had cancer and was
referred by her doctor because she had a "family
problem." Mrs. Myer and her siblings were financially
affluent but had relationships that resulted in constant bickering. She herself had a harsh, cold, punitive personality. The well-to-do 80-year-old father
maintained the family home and supervised in a slight-
ly doddering fashion a retarded 45-year-old sister
who had spent many years in institutions. The patient's
problem was her determination to make definite and
permanent arrangements with someone who would give
her an unbreakable guarantee that after her death
her sister would never be placed in an institution.
This, of course, was impossible to secure and no
other kind of help could reach the patient to modify
or alter her wishes in the slightest degree.

(b) Subjective vs. Objective Reality

Mr. Allore, age 34, his wife and two pre-school
children had emigrated to Canada four years previously. He immediately developed physical complaints
related to his digestive system, but many tests and
examinations revealed no pathology. He was an accoun-
tant in his homeland but could not meet the standards
for a similar job in Canada. Consequently, he undertook retraining in two government-sponsored courses,
he failed in both and the failure he blamed on his
physical illness and his inability to understand

English. Neither excuse was an objective evaluation:
he was not ill and he spoke and understood English
satisfactorily. In order to provide for the family,
Mrs. Allore enrolled in a secretarial course which
she completed; she found a position. Mr. Allore remained at home doing the housework and caring for
the children. As a result, family roles became re-
versed and normal cultural behaviour was contra-
dicted. The social worker, even though she understood the psychodynamics of the situation, could not
help Mr. Allore to function in a way that was more
satisfying to him and his family. He continued to
attend clinics, to complain and, in fact, to feel
ill and demand assurance that he could always get
financial assistance from a social agency should he
need it.

(c) The Runaways

      Mrs. Bowman was referred to the social worker
when she told a doctor in clinic that she was worried
about her two children. Every member of the Bowman
family demonstrated in some form what might be called
   the runaway syndrome. Mr. Bowman deserted his wife
and two children; Mrs. Bowman left jobs; both children ran away from foster homes or from whichever
parent was currently looking after them; and the
whole family moved their possessions so frequently
that it was literally impossible to know at any given
   moment where to find them. Many social workers
from various agencies had tried to help this family
but no one was successful in resolving any part of
any problem: marital, financial, delinquency, or
housing.

(d) A Wilderness around Her

      Mrs. Goshen, age 60, looked age 70, despite her
soft hair and beautiful complexion. She had many and
varied physical complaints and in her own estimation
was very sick. She complained that she was allergic
to dust, she had an ulcer, she had rheumatism, and
she had a swollen leg. The fact that only the varicosities were real did not deter her from coming to
several clinics every week. She was a deserted wife
(Mr. Goshen was now dead) and abandoned mother (the
whereabouts of her daughter, age 35, were unknown),

and she had estranged her only brother and his family.
She denied quarrelling with him and said that she
only told him what she thought. She bickered constantly with her landlady who complained that Mrs.
Goshen was too demanding. This picture had remained
constant for two years but neither person would take
any action: Mrs. Goshen refused to find other
accommodation and the landlady would not ask her to
leave. Mrs. Goshen felt entitled to her own apartment
(her only income was from public assistance), her
own television, and new clothes every season, as well
as pounds of pills from the out-patient department.
When all her demands were not met, she had a temper
tantrum with all the elements of a three-year-old
level of emotional development. Any and every attempt
at helping her to develop insight was fruitless;
her reply was: "I should be treated like a queen --
I'm a 'spectable woman."

At one point, her varicosities became so in-
flamed that she was admitted to hospital for a venal
ligation. She had decided it was not a convenient
time of year to be in hospital but was persuaded by
the nurse, the doctor, and two social workers that
this was indeed the time. However, she had such a
temper tantrum in the operating room and her blood
pressure became so elevated that the surgeon cancelled
the operation and Mrs. Goshen went home firmly convinced that she was critically ill and required a
winter in Florida.

She remains so demanding, so dissatisfied with
everything, and has such outbursts of crying and
whining that only a social worker with the stoutest
character can sustain the case for more than six
months. She involves secretaries, volunteers, other
patients and passers-by with her stories. Psychiatric
consultation confirmed a social worker's diagnosis
that she had a character disorder but psychiatric
skills could offer no help.

(e)   The Many Others

But these are not the only hearts that are dis-
tant and create wildernesses around themselves. The
alcoholics, the transients, the recurrent unmarried
mothers, the patients who have no available sense
of their own dignity are but some of those who cannot
or indeed who will not be helped. The files of every

social service department, of every social agency
contain a wide variety of case histories: some are
failures, some are successes. They are alike in
showing the infinite varieties of pathos, humour,
strength, and weakness that social workers find
themselves encountering.

CHAPTER IX

THE FUNCTIONS ARE MANY

"The Social Service Department provides
oil that enables the complicated hospital
machinery to move smoothly and efficiently,
assists the patients to have that peace of
mind that allows them to benefit to the
full from the medical and surgical care,
and provides the important liaison with the
community that results in good public relations and the most effective use of resources." [1]

In the preceding chapter examples were provided to
illustrate the social worker's function in direct
social work treatment. This is her major task and
absorbs most of her working time. Other aspects of
the department's activity -- such as administration,
supervision, staffing and programming must be performed efficiently within a solid structural framework. This same framework is needed to support the
workers as they perform other functions which are
also basic to effective social work treatment and
factors which assist in providing total and comprehensive care for the patient.

1. Appropriate Use of Community Resources

     The social worker can be a strong liaison
between the patient, the home, the hospital, and the
community, and her skills and techniques can be used
to return the patient to that part of the community
which will offer him care and most satisfaction for
his needs. Consequently, thorough knowledge of the
community's resources and how to use them appropriately is essential for medical social workers.

---

1. Avis Pumphrey, "Social Worker in a Hospital--Why?"
Canadian Welfare, Vol. 38, No. 5, p. 201 (Sept. 15,
1962).

The questions, what is a community and what is a resource, require broad answers. No longer does a community have only the narrow sense of a group or municipality. In our one world, it has expanded to include not only a province or a state or even a country; it may reach into every country on every continent. The ease, made possible by technology, with which individuals move from one place to another, has complicated the concept of community in a manner unknown before and many a social worker has personal evidence of this. Therefore a knowledge of when and how to use which international organizations, is at times as essential as knowing the when, which, and how of local or national resources.

The interesting experience of a worker in using the facilities of the International Social Service illustrates this. A 70-year-old man, with a coronary, was determined to fly the Atlantic and go to live with his daughter in southern France. Father and daughter had not met for 25 years and the worker did not know whether or not she wanted the father, or knew of his enfeebled condition or had any room for him; she even feared his being stranded at Orly airport. Consequently, she wrote the International Social Service (in triplicate), outlined the situation and asked them to have someone visit the daughter. The reply assured the worker of her patient's welcome but posed another problem. The patient's wife, whom he had last seen 40 years earlier in Bulgaria, was now living with her daughter too. When the patient learned this, he required the worker's help to sort out his feelings and to adjust to the idea of being a married man again. Finally, he decided to try it and left for France.

An appreciation of what is a resource is also vital. When a resource is needed, the search may extend not only to such facilities as organized agencies and institutions, but also to churches and church groups, government representatives at all levels, police, neighbours, auxiliaries of all kinds including those of the armed services, women's groups, benevolent associations, PTA organizations, service clubs, schools, and a plethora of others. Resources (there seems to be no other word that conveys the same meaning) are multiplying with great rapidity both geographically and governmentally. Communities are developing new ones every day, and are enacting

new legislation or modifying old. It is unrealistic
to think of teaching a student or expecting a worker
to know all the possible resources. However, it is
realistic to expect both staff and students to be
able to identify the kind of   resource that could
most appropriately be used to meet any given need,
and then to search for it. Of course, facility in
this technique is acquired only by practice and
experience. The social worker in the hospital must
thus have an ever-widening horizon and learn to use
professionally the resources of a one-world community
with precision, discretion and creativity. Perhaps
the last is the most important word.

     The greatest number of contacts with community
resources are made on direct behalf of a patient and/
or with his family with whom the worker is concerned,
but the worker's knowledge of what is available in
the community may also be used indirectly, for example, in consultation, when a doctor inquires about
housing facilities in a particular neighbourhood for
a patient he is treating in his office. There are
also occasions when a resource or a service may be
required by a member of the hospital staff, a doctor,
or the hospital itself. The need may become known to
the administrator, the head of any department, or
indeed anyone in the hospital. Often, hospital
personnel find themselves personally in problem situa-
tionsthat the use of a community resource might solve.
An example might be the ward aide whose paralysed
husband can no longer be left alone, the nurse who
needs a day nursery for her child, the orderly whose
son is delinquent, or the doctor whose elderly mother
requires nursing home care. An interesting gauge of
the level of understanding of social work may indeed
be how often a member of the hospital staff asks a
social worker for help with a personal problem or
for some specific information about the community.

2. Community Liaison

     This is a broad and perhaps somewhat nebulous
function. It is also one in which many if not all
hospital employees participate, if only from the
public relations aspect. Certainly an employee who
is happy in his job and speaks positively about the
hospital, even to a limited circle of relatives and

friends, is doing good public relations work. However, important as this contribution is, it of course
lacks the depth and productivity of the conscious
action that is required to help give a hospital its
place in a community structure. The walls that used
to isolate the hospital and its activities from the
public are tumbling down and exposing the hospital
to the community and the community to the hospital.
If these changes are to be constructive, interpretation of each to the other must take place constantly,
and the social workers have an obligation to participate   by interpreting the hospital and its services to the community and the needs and plans of the
community to the hospital.
    There are many ways in which social workers can
do this. One might be the giving of a paper or a speech,
or the writing of an article for publication -- tasks
which might seem daunting to some but which fulfil a
service to hospital and profession. Perhaps the most
common method is active participation in health and
welfare committees that are community-based. Medical
social workers should indeed be expected to assume
responsibility in such committees as part of their
job. Undoubtedly some committees meet endlessly and
achieve nothing. But these are exceptions. Careful
selection of committees, those that are sponsored by
the profession of social work and those under the
aegis of community groups, and appropriate and continuing involvement in their work will mean better
liaison between the hospital and the community.
    Opportunities for community liaison present them-
selves in other ways. Sometimes a worker becomes aware
of some hostility or rejection of the   hospital's
patients by another organization, and when she does
she must do something about it. A worker was once told
by the admitting clerk of a convalescent hospital that
she didn't want to take her patient because the worker's hospital didn't follow the convalescent hospital
rules. Further discussion revealed that the convalescent hospital required that every patient there be
visited at least once a week by his private physician,
and doctors from the worker's hospital refused to make
such visits. This information was given by the worker
to her director and by her to the Chief of Staff who
brought it to the attention of all services at a
Medical Advisory Council Meeting.
    To take another example of community liaison.

The supervisor of an Unmarried Parents Department of a Children's Aid Society called the director of social service because a number of unmarried mothers whose babies had been placed for adoption became upset when they were visited by a public health nurse "to see the baby." The director traced these situations until she found how and where the mistake was being made. A recently employed clerk who was responsible for sending the Department of Health notification of all births had not understood that such referrals did not include mothers whose babies died or were placed in foster homes by a social agency.

3. Information and Help in Formulating Social Policies and Procedures Affecting Patients and Staff

There are many areas in the hospital in which routines or procedures are adhered to long after the reason for their existence has been forgotten and their usefulness has disappeared. These may affect not only patients but staff, and may militate against intelligent care of the patient and lower staff morale. Every hospital has these uneasy areas, and the administrator who believes his hospital is free of them should rush for help. The social worker has some liaison with virtually every department, and she may by this fact alone be able to see the ramifications of inadequate policies and the overlooking of ones that are not being honoured.

An example might be the situation where a new policy about admitting hours was made and patients were told to be in the hospital for admission between the hours of 12:30 and 2:00 p.m.; the result was that the admitting clerks were overwhelmed, delayed their lunch hours or didn't have any lunch and, consequently, became irritable both with patients and one another. The patients, some of them miserably ill and in pain, and all of them becoming increasingly anxious, waited an unnecessarily long time. The situation came to the attention of the social workers when two of the patients known to them became very upset and one went home refusing to be admitted at all. At this point, the director discussed the policy with the administrator and contributed to formulating a new policy and procedure that was satisfactory to all the departments involved, and more conducive to the

comfort of the patient. Social work skills and techniques may also be used when policies or procedures
are being established or changed that are related to
fee schedules, reports to agencies, automatic referrals to visiting nurse organizations, or which involve the social well-being of the patient in any
way. It is characteristic of a social worker by definition that she listens to people who are having difficulty or who are dissatisfied, and because of this,
she may become aware of trouble spots.

The above does not mean, of course, that the
social workers are the only people who are likely
to be aware of trouble spots in the organization; it
only means that because of their particular skills
in the understanding of behaviour and their contacts
with a cross-section of the hospital population, they
are a valuable resource to administration in helping
oil the organizational machinery. Nor should it carry
any implication that this activity be done either on
the basis of gossip on one hand or spying on the
other. It is a simple statement of the real fact that
social workers have a knowledge of human problems
and techniques to understand the cause of social dysfunction and may know a method of resolution.

4. Staff Teaching

Teaching is a definite function of the Social
Service Department and should be recognized as such.
Arrangements can be made for it to be done on a
formal basis when a course is concerned with the
social aspects of illness. Every hospital, whether
or not it is affiliated with a university, contains
within its functions that of teaching. Sometimes
this function is formal and designated persons carry
recognized roles as teachers; sometimes it is indirect
and even haphazard so that although teaching is done
in many ways, it is done without a label. A positive
climate toward education is determined both by the
general attitude of the hospital administration and
by that of the department itself. In a broad hospital
program, social work teaching about the social component of illness would be included as part of the
in-service education of all professional staff. The
kind of material taught must, of course, be geared

to the needs of those being taught; for example, the
dietitian requires a different level of understanding
from that of the nurse, the intern a different one
from that of the experienced physician.

It was noted in Chapter V (page 43) that some
faculties of medicine provide adequate instruction
in this subject and the students from medical schools
which have a social worker on their staff develop
not only an appreciation of the social component of
illness, but are better able to perceive the sick as
people. With young doctors, the hospital social
worker's role is greatly lessened. It may be, however,
that the lecturer who has been assigned to teach a
course on the social aspects of illness has had little
preparation and not much experience in using the subject matter. Too often, the social component of illness is taught not by a social worker, but by a
sociologist, psychologist or even a member of the medical
profession to students in the same profession. As a
result of teaching done in this manner, the students
will not gain enough knowledge or understanding, and
may even develop a negative attitude that such things
are not very pertinent as far as their own professional education is concerned. Then, again, it does
seem to be true that doctors are becoming more and
more concerned with the science of medicine and with
methods of treatment the results of which can be
scientifically proven and less concerned with the
personal speciality of the patient. In the past ten
or twelve years, doctors have, indeed, written a
great many books and articles(to be found in both
public and professional libraries), the main theme
of which has been a re-emphasis on the humanity of
the patient. In a series of articles entitled "Our
Doctor Dilemma" a junior intern was quoted: "today,
people being attracted to medicine are more scientifically than humanistically oriented." [2] Perhaps,
in 1893, Goldwin Smith had a premonition of what
would happen to people in a technocracy when he said:
"a romantic age stands in need of science, a scientific age stands in need of the humanities." [3]

---

2. "Our Doctor Dilemma," Toronto Daily Star, March
20, 1967, p. 3.

3. Goldwin Smith, quoted in the newspaper The Week,
April 28, 1893, published in Toronto.

It is essential today that the hospital deliberately provide structured educational experiences for its staff about the humanity of men.

(a) <u>Interns and Residents</u>. Social work teaching for interns and residents to be most profitable might well begin on the day of their orientation to the hospital by a meeting with the Director of Social Work. However, because of the general excitement that usually prevails at this time, only a few facts can then be presented and assimilated. Perhaps the only fact that will be retained is that administration recognizes social work as part of patient care, and it is of sufficient significance to be included in their first day's experience. Further lectures and discussion periods should be included in their lecture schedule during the year. Undoubtedly, how much beginning doctors are able to take into consideration beyond the lab reports is in direct relation to their basic personal human responses which determine whether or not they are able to practise medicine both as an art and a science, or as a science alone.

(b) <u>Staff Doctors</u>. Staff doctors who have been in practice many years vary in their acceptance of the significance of their patients' social problems. Usually the general practitioner, by the nature of his professional activities, is more attuned to the social needs of his patients than the specialist, who may often seem to feel that his job and interest in the patient are limited to the diseased part with which his specialty is concerned. The following illustration is a striking example of this, but it should be stressed that it is not meant as a generalization but an indication of possible danger in situations where specialists are particularly involved.

When a 54-year-old woman, who had been in hospital for six months following a double leg amputation, was ready for transfer to a long-term care hospital she was referred back to her family physician. He learned that the other hospital had extra charges for certain services and because he was uncertain whether his patient had any financial resources, referred the patient to the social worker. The money was no problem, but nobody had noticed that the patient had lost herself. Her ego image had been damaged, she could see nothing for herself in the future, and

she questioned who and what she was in the present.
She had been a "cooperative" patient and, in being
so, had become frightened and withdrawn and repeated
over and over to the worker: "But what about me --
what about me?" not so much as a query as a statement.
The point of the story is apparent.

There are several methods of informing staff
doctors about the social implications of illness but
it is obvious that they cannot be utilized unless
they have the support of either or both the members
of the Medical Advisory Council and individual chiefs
of staff. If a chief is willing, the program of a
full staff meeting of his specialty once a year could
be on social work. Social work ward rounds on a regularly scheduled basis with case discussion following
is another method. Other ways and means can be developed according to the skills of the director and the
collaboration of the doctors. 4

(c) <u>Nurses and Others</u>. Many schools of nursing,
especially those affiliated with medical schools,
have established courses on the social aspect of the
patient, but as in medical schools, these may be
taught by nurses, sociologists or psychologists, and
whether or not the material becomes smothered by the
skills of nursing as such is likely to be determined
by the personality of the student nurse. It is then
possible that patients might only be regarded as
being co-operative or unco-operative, which means:
do they require a great deal of attention, do they
cry, rather than why are they frightened.

4. In the report of his study on <u>The General Pract-
itioner</u> Kenneth Clute outlines his criteria for evaluating "a very good history." According to his assess-
ment, histories are "very good" if they include the
doctor's investigation of the possibility of complica-
tions, differential diagnoses, and major organ systems other than the one related to the patient's complaints. However, he makes no reference even by in-
ference to the social situation, the patient's family,
or possible emotional involvement or reaction. <u>The
General Practitioner</u>: <u>A Study of Medical Education
and Practice in Ontario and Nova Scotia</u> (University
of Toronto Press), p. 266.

In hospitals where there are both social service
departments and schools of nursing, introduction to
the human side of the patients with all their problems and successes, their joys, sorrows and fears,
should be taught by a social worker before the nursing students have their first ward experience. The
nurse who becomes a supervisor without this kind of
learning might set a climate on her ward that pro-
hibits the full co-operation of her nursing staff
with the doctors and the social workers simply because she has not been taught in a vital way the
larger concept of the patient. Often, of course, a
nurse may have an intuitive way of responding positively to the human needs of her patients, but she
would be better equipped to do so constructively if
she had some of the learning referred to here.

There are other hospital staff who have direct
contact with patients who need this same kind of
learning experience. These include dietitians,
physical and occupational therapists, and lab tech-
nicians.

(d) Students. The teaching of students does not
relate only to those in social work, but may well include any student or group of students for whom the
hospital provides an educational experience, i.e.
medical students, hospital administration students,
dietetic students and others. The teaching program
should be adapted to the specific professional needs.

Social work students are a particular responsibility of any department whose professional standards meet the requirements of a school of social
work. However, such students should be accepted only
when there is sufficient staff to carry the work load
of the department, so that the field instructor will
have adequate time to give her students the teaching
and help they require.

The social work student should be in the second
year of the master's program. The first year student,
unless there are extenuating circumstances, has not
usually had time to be sufficiently at ease in her
new helping role to adjust and to cope with the
pressures of the crises in illness. These pressures
are accentuated for her by the presence of the whole
range of hospital personnel, all working within their
own different frameworks of job responsibility, but

with whom the student must collaborate.

Field instruction for students in social work is a method with a twofold purpose. It provides an opportunity for them to integrate theory and to see results in a concrete, visible way which will enable them later to apply their skills and techniques appropriately and flexibly. Also, it demonstrates to the field instructor and through her to the school authorities whether or not the students concerned are the kind of people who are able to sustain, within a professional identity, the emotional demands that are so heavy in the practice of the social work profession.

The costs, usually hidden, of student teaching are high but the returns are usually high too, to the department and subsequently to hospital and patients. The exchange of knowledge and experience between the social work field consultant and the field instructor should be shared with the whole staff so that they will be stimulated to increase their own professional competence. The contact with a university faculty demands that standards be scrutinized regularly and the sharpening of the skills needed in teaching provides better supervisory skills which result in a better quality of patient care. Also, there is the very good practical reason that the more students who have medical social work training, the more workers will be available to fill social work positions in hospitals. If money for bursaries can be located (perhaps from the Women's Auxiliary), and given for social work education to a student interested in a commitment to medical social work, professionally trained staff will be augmented.

CHAPTER X

SOCIAL WORK: THE THIRD DIMENSION

"In poverty I lack other things...
in sickness I lack myself." 1

The hospital (any hospital) is a fascinating world
in itself, with a complicated structure carefully
arranged around a designated purpose, a hierarchy
of staff, a budget, established policies and procedures; all have been conditioned, of course, by
time and custom. The hospital is also an instrument
of the society in which it exists and as such is
committed to provide the best possible care and
treatment for the sick of that society. It is a pro-
vocative and sobering thought that patients and their
families still expect the same services of care and
comforting, of treatment and healing that they did
fifty, forty, or even ten years ago, and do so in
spite of all the sophistications of medical care
produced by technocracy and even by the welfare
state which, in less than a generation, have radically
changed ways of life and many values. Perhaps this
expectation is rooted in an uneasy feeling that money
and material objects are not in themselves enough.
Perhaps it is because it is the human condition to
need individual care if healing is to occur. Perhaps
it is because "the stressfulness of illness and medical care is beyond the adjustive capacity of many
individuals." 2 For all of these and a variety of
other reasons, social work with its particular focus
on the needs and capacities of individuals is required to provide the third dimension to patient
care.
     The hospital as a corporate body is in a con-
stant state of change and every year becomes more

1. John Donne, Sermon XX.

2. Harriet M. Bartlett, "The Widening Scope of Hospital Social Work," Journal of Social Case Work (Published by the National Association of Social Workers,

complex both in its administration and in the obli-
gations it assumes in the community in which it is
set. In the last two decades, it has begun and will
continue to be more and more like a business institution with the inevitable power struggles between the
financing body, board, administration, medical and
other professional staff and, indeed, the community.
The community indeed now perceives the hospital as
its own, and the more widespread pre-paid hospital
and doctor insurance coverage becomes, the more will
people become concerned, in a variety of attitudes,
with the services of the hospital. Working amid all
these stresses and strains, the hospital does provide
an ever increasing and better quality of care for the
physically and mentally ill because of the application of many developments in medical and allied
sciences, and by including social work in its complement of services, it is enabled to apply a humanistic philosophy that recognizes and honours the
humanity of its patients.
        One of the fathers of modern medicine, Sir
William Osler, gave particular emphasis to the in-
dividuality of patients and throughout his lectures
and writings he returned frequently to the importance
of knowing the patient. This philosophy is found in
almost every paper included in Aequanimitas and Other
Addresses and it is epitomized in his address "Books
and Men" delivered at the Boston Medical Library in
1901. He says: "to study the phenomena of disease
without books is to sail an uncharted sea, while to
study bodies without the patient is not to go to sea
at all." 3 In reading Aequanimitas, it is impossible
not to recognize how Osler emphasized two aspects in
the practice of medicine: one he called "the leaven
of science" and the other "the art of practice."
In "Leaven of Science," an address given at the open-
ing of the Wistar Institute of Anatomy and Biology,
Philadelphia,in 1894, he says,"science has done much
and will do more" but in the same paragraph he continues, "with reason science never parts company,
but with feeling, emotion, passion, what has she to
do? They are not of her; they owe her no allegiance.

New York) Vol. 8, No. 1, 1963, p. 6.

3. Sir William Osler, Aequanimitas and Other Addresses,
3rd ed. (Philadelphia, Blakiston 1945), p. 210.

She may study, analyse and define, she can never
control them and by no possibility can their ways
be justified to her." [4] By emphasizing the human
emotions and feelings of the patient, Osler nevertheless did not move science and the scientific
method from their place in the treatment of disease.
But it is reasonable to assume that he could not anti-
cipate the full development of technology nor its
effect on the practice of medicine. No one would be
without the continuous discoveries of science, and
yet they have now made it very difficult for all individual doctors to know and understand all that is
available to be known and to develop the necessary
skills to use the new knowledge in even a very
specialized segment of their own profession and still
keep the personalities of patients in adequate view.

In order to test how Osler's teachings had
survived in modern medical practice, I once did a
most non-scientific sampling, of no design whatever,
with about two dozen doctors among whom were chiefs
of service, junior and senior attending staff, and
residents and interns. The only constants in this
sample were the fact that I knew each of these men
personally and that they all had a degree in medicine.
I simply asked them, "What do you think of Osler's
philosophy of patient care?" Some hesitated before
replying, realizing that it was a loaded question.
Others answered immediately and the answer, with one
exception, was along these lines: "He is old-fashioned,"
"he is not scientific," "modern medicine cannot be
practised as he taught," "there isn't time to do what
he wanted done"; most of them added: "Medicine is a
science now." The one exception was a junior intern
who said with obvious embarrassment: "I'd like to be
more interested in the person but the scientific
demands on me are too great."

Illness has many forms and undoubtedly many
meanings. How the patient perceives his illness can
often only be understood in relation to his culture,
sub-culture, social class, religion, ego image and
libidinal needs and the methods by which he makes
his social adaptations. This understanding needs to
be made evident in a positive transaction if the

------

4. Ibid., p. 93.

sick person is to make maximal use of medical and
nursing care and so be able to return to an optimal
level of physical and social functioning. However,
social work cannot claim to be able to cure all the
heart aches or relieve all the social problems in-
digenous to the human condition, any more than the
hospitals in which it is practised can offer any
promise that all patients will be made physically
whole or that every patient will be discharged alive.
The social work profession has to recognize its own
inadequacies, the lacunae in its knowledge, the im-
perfections of its techniques and the limitations of
the material with which it works. But like every
other profession whose discipline is sincere, it must
try constantly to enlarge its horizons, its knowledge,
and its potential for giving help, and therefore must
attempt to re-identify its role and functions in an
effort to keep them in alignment with the needs of
the people whom it serves.

Social work must, then, always strive to become
more flexible. It should also endeavour to be sufficiently secure in itself so that it may become more
comfortable in sharing the process of social treatment. Social workers know that social work is often
confusing to those outside the profession and that
others find it difficult to understand that a professional discipline has arisen whose sole goal is to
help people in trouble by the use of a relationship.
People are people; everybody has troubles; everybody
has relationships; everybody (consciously or unconsciously) helps somebody else. The obvious question is: "what's so special about that?" But everybody also experiences health and sickness, and everybody has a personal remedy for every ill. Sometimes
these home-grown methods are effective, sometimes
they are not, and when they fail, the expert skill
of the doctor is required. Just so, every social mal-
adjustment does not need to be, and indeed could not
be, treated by a social worker. However, when friend-
ly counselling fails, the competence of the social
worker in using relationship with constructive deli-
beration and within the reality of the person-problem
complex often achieves a return to a level of social
health that could not otherwise be reached. Inevitably, of course, in some situations and with some
people, social work must fail since social workers

are human, social agencies are organized by humans, and some human social illnesses are malignant and terminal.

One of the major problems of today is the tendency of the individual to be lost in the mass, and the unhappy consciousness of this on his part. The feeling is intensified when a person becomes a patient and gives himself over to the complexities of modern medicine. This almost universal emotion of "aloneness" can be further intensified by a sociological determinant expressed in an attitude of current society that feelings or reactions of dependency and hostility are not permissible or acceptable. To feel or express either emotion can often be considered by our pseudo-sophisticated society to be signs of a failure. Everyone is expected to be capable of controlling and managing his life without any allowance being made for human fraility or the occurrence of a catastrophe beyond his control. However, when a person becomes ill and has physical symptoms of illness, a certain limited acceptance of social failure and dependency is forthcoming. It is then that it becomes socially acceptable to admit the presence of social problems and it is at these times that, if the social worker's help is offered, it can be accepted.

The problems with which patients need help run the whole gamut of human experience. For some, a solution is readily available and eagerly accepted by the individuals involved. For others, a solution must not only be found but offered in such a way that it can be used in whole or in part by the troubled person. For still others no solution is possible. Always the social worker must see the whole patient, his problem, his life experience, his potential in their cultural, social, and psychological dimensions. Ida Cannon, in an address before the American Hospital Association in October, 1920, spoke these words no less true in 1968: "The social worker's biggest contribution to the hospital [is] that of never thinking in routine, of keeping fresh always the community's and the patient's point of view." Hospitals are for patients and if the patient focus should be lost, hospitals cannot justify their costly existence. Social work is for the individual and medical social work is particularly for the individual who is sick.

Social work, based as it is on a belief in the value of the individual as a human, social, emotional, and spiritual being, has thus a deep and great contribution to make in relation to applied science. If this contribution is to be effective in the hospital organization and in the care of the patient, understanding of it by the hospital authority, the doctors, and the nurses is essential. Social work needs no apologia for its place in the hospital organization, but it does need a broader understanding of why it has a place and full acknowledgement of its place. Hospitals that include a well functioning, professionally oriented social service department will not hear the cry of their patients in the words of John Donne: "In poverty I lack other things... in sickness I lack myself."

ADDITIONAL BACKGROUND REFERENCES

Books

1. Arthur C. Bachmeyer M.D., and Gerhard Hartman Ph.D.,
   The Hospital in Modern Society (New York: The
   Commonwealth Fund, 1943).

2. Richard C. Cabot M.D., Social Service and the Art
   of Healing (New York: Moffat, Yard & Co., 1909).

3. Nathaniel W. Faxon M.D., The Hospital in Con-
   temporary Life (Cambridge: Harvard University
   Press, 1949).

4. Elizabeth A. Ferguson, Social Work: An Introduction
   (Philadelphia and New York: J.B. Lippincott Co.,
   1963).

5. Eliot Friedson, Editor, The Hospital in Modern
   Society, (Toronto: Collier-Macmillan Canada Ltd.,
   1963).

6. Celia Moss, Administering a Hospital Social Service
   Department (Washington: American Association of
   Medical Social Workers, 1955).

Articles

1. Edna Osborne, "The Social Worker's Expanding Role
   in Continuity of Care," The Social Worker, April-
   May, 1964 (Canadian Association of Social Workers,
   Ottawa).

2. "Educational Qualifications of Medical Social
   Workers in Public Health Programs," American
   Journal of Public Health, Vol. 48, No. 8.

3. "Esssntial Elements in Education for Medical
   Social Workers," Medical Social Work, 1950.